THE MOON AND MADNESS

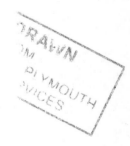

THE MOON AND MADNESS

Niall McCrae

imprint-academic.com

Published in the UK by Imprint Academic
PO Box 200, Exeter EX5 5YX, UK

Published in the USA by Imprint Academic
Philosophy Documentation Center
PO Box 7147, Charlottesville, VA 22906-7147, USA

ISBN 9 781845 42143

A CIP catalogue record for this book is available from the
British Library and US Library of Congress

Contents

Tables

Dr Paul Crawford

Foreword

A certain woman, named Leviva, from Wrokestan (a vill[age] near Banbury), suffered continually for three years from a swelling of the womb so that her body became useless with the anxiety and pain. Eventually she became so heavily weighed down with humours that she was unable to work. Her womb was inflated to such an extent that her neighbours said she presented the appearance of someone pregnant. Her clothes scarcely fitted her. The swelling spread to the rest of her body, even her hands and feet, and was worse at full moon. She said that this malady came on through the bitter cold when she went to the toilet, so that sometimes she made canine barking noises. She was judged mad (*vesania*) by everyone and tied up. Because of this she was rejected by her husband. She went to the church of the blessed virgin, and persisted in the most devoted prayer throughout the night. After much pain and trembling, with belching and yawning, she was freed from the noxious humours with which she had been impregnated, and her health returned.

'Miracula S. Frideswidae', *Acta Sanctorum Bollandiana*,
VIII Oct. (Antwerp, 1853), 27: 574

In the Miracles of St Frideswide in the medieval period we find a captivating narrative of Leviva who becomes 'barking mad' under the influence of the full moon yet recovers miraculously after praying through the night. This link between the full moon and transformation or transmogrification into a mad, moonstruck or dangerous 'other', most notably a werewolf, has featured prominently from the classical the writings of Herodotus, Virgil or Ovid to Kipling's *Mark of the Beast*, Beaugrand's *The Werwolves* or more recent popular fiction such as Patricia Briggs' *Moon Called* or Jim Butcher's *Fool Moon*. Lychanthropy (transformation into a wolf) has also made it into many films, not least *Werewolf of London*, *The Howling*, *Mad at the Moon* or as Fenrir Greyback and Remus Lupin in the Harry Potter films. We can even listen to Ozzy Osbourne howling in 'Bark at the Moon' or the slightly more lyrical 'Full Moon' by The Kinks:

Haven't you noticed a kind of madness in my eyes?
It's only me, dear, in my midnight disguise.
Pay no attention if I crawl across the room.
It's just another full moon.
Don't be afraid of me when I'm walking in my sleep.
Don't get alarmed, dear, when I start to crawl and creep.
Try not to listen when I mumble like a loon.
It's just another full moon.
It's just another full moon.

In folklore, literature, film and music, the werewolf as cultural product has emerged from the various threats, imagined or real, that humans have faced, mixing the wolf as feared nocturnal predator with other disturbing phenomena or beliefs, be it seizures or unpredictable behaviour, unexplained deaths, serial killings, mutilations, the Devil or other evil spirits. In short, this particular shape-shifter has been associated with being possessed, murderous, odd-looking or mad. Thus strong candidates for being considered werewolves in the past were individuals suffering psychosis, or those with conditions such as Down's Syndrome, congenital porphyria (comprising psychosis and reddened teeth), rabies, epilepsy or hypertrichosis (excessive or abnormal hair growth). Indeed, individuals suffering delusions about being an animal or able to transform into an animal (clinical lychanthropy) may well have assisted processes of social exclusion and stigmatisation.

Howling at the moon has certainly been an enduring image down the ages and the full moon has long been associated with provoking madness. Yet, in this age of evidence-based everything, it remains to be seen whether the archaic and largely obsolete notion of *lunacy* (referring to an intermittent insanity under the influence of the full moon) will be seriously revisited as a phenomenon. One wonders if the sheer appetite for fantasy literature that continues to this day, the demand for stories about vampires and werewolves, is part of the problem here. The constant revisiting in the imagination and unending representations in popular culture of the transformation into a werewolf under the light of the moon could well be one of the reasons why lunar influence is not taken seriously.

Niall McCrae's book offers a fascinating account of the history of claims about the moon's influence on us and suggests that conflicting evidence on this should not mean an end to the investigation. Importantly, McCrae's book presents a sober overview of the development of ideas about the relationship between the universe and humankind, and an as yet inconclusive inquiry into the physics that might support the long held belief that our satellite pulls on or otherwise disturbs the balance of our minds and bodies.

Drawing upon theories from Ancient times to the present day, McCrae brings the cosmos to life. We sense its material and trajectory. We get to see our own planet as something fragile and pliable, and empathize with those complex, water-clothed skeletons moving about on its crust. We begin to acknowledge the play of gravity and light in the universe. We consider magnetism and how it makes iron filings stand up like hairs on the neck or guides migrating birds. And we begin to suspect that alongside the magical and puzzling realm of sub-atomic particles or dark matter, clouds giving birth to distant stars and our own sun spitting at us from time to time that we face all kinds of pulls and pushes, all kinds of unfelt caresses beyond the movement of air. Who is to say that we are not worked on by the moon in a similar way to our oceans or prodded by its light into a restless sleep that brings out the wolf in us? As the author notes in his concluding remarks, phenomena appear to correlate with the moon's cycles: 'Beans spurt, sea urchins bulge, worms glow, clams open, wolves howl. What theoretical obstacle precludes human sensitivity to the perturbations of our satellite?'

In his concluding remarks, McCrae argues for an alchemy of interpretative and positivist (scientific) research into the influence of the moon on mental state, observing a major fault-line in contemporary psychiatry: its privileging of knowledge that has little to do with richer human experience and narratives. Contemporary psychiatry, he suggests, remains heavily fixated on outcome measurements. McCrae is not alone in identifying this shortfall. A number of critics, most recently Richard Bentall, have seriously questioned the foundations of its practice. In reading this book one is left wondering whether psychiatry and its preferred evidence base, as in the lyrics by the Waterboys, might be seeing 'the crescent' rather than the 'whole of the moon.' Equally, one might wonder about the kind of rationality on offer in psychiatry and science generally and question the madness in its method, rather as the great eighteenth-century painter Joseph Wright of Derby did. Although not officially a member of the Lunar Society, or 'lunatick', Wright was keen to study the play of light and in particular moonlight. In his disturbing work, *An Experiment on a Bird in the Air Pump*, held at the National Gallery, London, he portrays a 'mad-scientist' demonstrating the creation of a vacuum that suffocates a bird. It is no coincidence that through the window to the right of the canvas, we see a full moon emerging from behind a cloud.

Dr Paul Crawford
Professor of Health Humanities
University of Nottingham

Preface

Bleary-eyed in the crisp dawn light of five minutes to seven, I paced along the glazed-brick corridor toward Cedar Ward, in the hinterland of a Victorian mental hospital. My arrival at the nurses' station drew little response from night staff concentrating on their final task before handover, muttering as they scribbled, each completed patient's record added to a stack on the desk. Then charge nurse Archie breezed in, punctuating the writing frenzy. 'That was one hell of a shift', exclaimed June; 'They've been up all night, going berserk — one after the other'. Details emerged of an early hours verbal joust between Albert and Lizzie, Kristos repeatedly wandering naked from his dormitory and high-pitched expletives from Martha about an alleged nocturnal theft, the rumpus culminating in Terry lashing out at Albert and Lizzie being banished to the quiet room after tearing curtains from the rail.[1] Remarkably to me, these events were collectively blamed on the full moon.

As a psychiatric nurse trainee enthused by the technical discourse around mental illness and its treatment, I found the notion of moon-forged madness difficult to take seriously. Yet these narrators were not Cub Scouts on camp regaling ghost stories, each scarier than the last. In my itinerant career in mental health services I have met numerous colleagues who have observed in patients a susceptibility to lunar provocation. Carmel, for example, who worked for thirty years at Netherne Mental Hospital in Surrey, recalled a consensus amongst nurses that wards were more chaotic at full moon, with sceptical novices soon convinced by experience. Such belief, I discovered, was not confined to psychiatric settings. My sister, a midwife in a prestigious central London maternity hospital, works with many colleagues who insist that full moon is a trigger for the breaking of waters.

---

1   All names have been changed in this anecdote.

Outside the healthcare setting, beliefs in the power of the Moon are not difficult to find. Rowan, barman of my local tavern, has observed lunar patterns in the mood of certain regulars. The most obvious case is an affable tradesman, who is normally to be found engaging in mundane chatter on weather, business and football. Occasionally, typically on his second pint, this customer's behaviour suddenly changes; his voice sharpens, and he becomes irritable and intolerant towards the idiosyncrasies of others — hardly a Transylvanian metamorphosis, but enough to make fellow drinkers wary. On heading home on these nights, Rowan has consistently found the carpark bathed in full moonlight. A retired fireman told me of a normally competent senior officer whose demeanour was known to change at full moon, when he became so confrontational that the men would steer clear of his path. These alleged 'turns' are but two examples relayed to me while writing this book. Uncritical acceptance of what some would suspect as the product of suggestion or selective recall will not be found in these pages, but nor should such observations be too readily dismissed. There is plenty of fantasy about the Moon, but here we are concerned with theory and evidence. Ultimately the reader will judge whether lunar influence on behaviour is real, possible or imagined.

Acknowledgements

Several people deserve my gratitude for their help with this project. For my initial inspiration in the field of mental health I would like to thank Jack Radcliffe Lyttle, my tutor at Argyll & Clyde College of Nursing. Charlie Russell, sadly deceased, was my mentor in mental health practice, and a key informant for this book. Michaela Poppe translated important German texts, proofread chapters many times, and gave valued comments. For hints on all matters astronomical, I thank my good friends James Gordon and especially Alan Morgan for his illuminations on electromagnetism. Alastair Macdonald helped to refine my critique of psychiatry. Rowan Barrett is owed a pint of bitter for his insightful observations on the real and paranormal world. I met Professor Paul Crawford at his conference on madness and literature at the University of Nottingham, where I first formally presented this work. I am immensely grateful to Paul for his substantial guidance on structure and content. Last but not least, I thank Catherine for her patience and support throughout.

Note on the text

The text follows the convention of using upper case for the Moon as a proper noun, and lower case when referring to the stages of lunar cycle (e.g. full moon).

Introduction

Th'unwearied sun from day to day
Does his Creator's pow'r display ...
Soon as the ev'ning shades prevail
The moon takes up the wondrous tale,
And nightly to the list'ning earth,
Repeats the story of her birth

Ode, Joseph Addison (1672–1719)

Our mystical Moon has long been an object of fantasy. The idea of lunar influence on behaviour can be traced back to antiquity, when people devised a myriad of supernatural explanations for the bewildering forces of nature. From centuries of careful observation, celestial patterns were deciphered, as humankind began to unravel the mysteries of the cosmos. Eventually the nocturnal beacon was deconsecrated from its heavenly throne, its goddesses starved by agnostic minds. Two millennia ago, it was realised that the transformation from acute crescent to disc was not due to shapeshifting, but light reflected at varying angles from the Sun. Through the telescopic endeavour of the Scientific Revolution, the *mare*, once thought to be seas, were revealed as desert plains. The 'dark side of the Moon' was reduced to an anthropic notion, our satellite being equally illuminated on its monthly rotation, and in 1959 photographs of the obscured face were obtained by the Russian craft *Luna 3*. Then, in July 1969, humankind had the impiety to tread on the garden of Selene. Any lingering notions of sentient lunar life were dispelled by probe samples, from which the Moon was determined as a barren rock, devoid of atmosphere. After *Apollo 11* there were further landings by NASA astronauts, but the race against the Soviet Union had been won, and with little prospect of viable human habitation, since 1972 the dust has settled on our lunar rambling (inevitably we will return, if only for mineral pillage).

In modern, urbanised society our satellite is sadly neglected, its luminary fluctuations noticed only as a curb to the enthusiasm of back-garden astronomers. Yet the Moon continues to inspire poet, philosopher and pagan alike, while for scientists it harbours truths yet untold. In a nineteenth-century theory, the Moon began as an enormous chunk thrown off by the rapid spinning motion of Earth, the resulting chasm now bathed by the Pacific Ocean. The problem with this idea is that lunar rock is of lower density than the crust of Earth. Another conjecture was of a roving body captured by Earth's gravitational field, but for this to happen without devastating collision is considered improbable. The most plausible genesis, as presented by astronomers William Hartmann and Donald Davis in the journal *Icarus* in 1975, is of a massive impact shortly after Earth was formed. In this account the young planet was struck by one of several huge lumps of molten rock in its vicinity, and the resulting debris condensed into a sphere. However, recent discovery of subterranean ice has raised doubts, as it had been assumed that the intense heat produced by the impact would have destroyed any volatile substances. The Moon is not so dead after all. All celestial bodies are in perpetual motion, and the relative aspect of Sun, Moon and Earth is constantly changing. There are consequently several lunar cycles, defined by point of reference. The synodic cycle is the circling of Earth by the Moon in relation to the Sun, and lasts an average of twenty-nine days, twelve hours and forty-four minutes. The period begins when the Moon is directly between Earth and the Sun, its illuminated side facing away from us. Full moon occurs a fortnight later when the Moon is on the opposite side of Earth from the Sun, so that a full disc is lit from our perspective. The sidereal cycle is the average of twenty-seven days, seven hours and forty-three minutes taken by the Moon to orbit Earth in relation to the stars. The synodic cycle is longer due to the progress of Earth around the Sun, requiring a little extra time for the Moon to complete its revolution. The waxing moon of first quarter is already high above the horizon at sunset, and sets about midnight. Full moon rises at sunset and disappears from view towards dawn. At third quarter the Moon is not seen until midnight, reaching its highest point at sunrise, and remaining visible well into daylight. Eclipses occur at syzygy, which means the exact alignment of three or more spheres in the same gravitational system. Due to the immense difference in size and distance, lunar eclipses, when sunlight casts the shadow of Earth on the Moon, are common, while solar eclipses are relatively rare events.

As well as its luminary prominence, the Moon exerts a constant, invisible force on the mother planet. In the universal law of gravitation revealed in the seventeenth century by Isaac Newton, mass attracts other mass relative to size and distance. Earth has a mass eighty times greater than the Moon, and the lunar pull is only 0.165 of the corresponding power of Earth. Terrestrial gravity has grossly distorted the lunar sphere, causing a bulge on its near face; as if in retaliation, the Moon has flattened the poles on Earth. As Earth spins, the seas closest to the Moon are pulled upwards. Land also rises; at the equator, by as much as fifty centimetres. Due to the orbit of Earth, high tides are twelve hours and twenty-five minutes apart, thus the lunar day is fifty minutes longer than the solar day. As the Moon's appearance on the horizon has a similar daily shift, a connection was long suspected, but not until Newton's *Principia* was this understood.

Apart from the daily rhythm, two principal factors modulate the tides. Firstly, there is the relative position of Sun and Moon. Twice each month, the tides rise furthest up the shore. These are the spring tides, and occur at new moon and full moon, when Sun and Moon are directly in line with Earth, and their gravitational force is combined (the tidal effect is delayed by a few days).[1] At first and third quarters, the pull of the Sun neutralises that of the Moon, resulting in the weaker neap tides of half moon. The second factor in tidal magnitude is the anomalistic cycle, which describes the distance of the Moon from Earth. This cycle has an average duration of twenty-seven days, thirteen hours and eighteen minutes, with extremes at apogee and perigee, when the Moon is furthest and nearest to Earth respectively. Tidal range is greatest when new or full moon corresponds with perigee. The extent of ebb and flow also varies from one part of a coast to another, due to local topography; the highest range, at an average of twelve metres, is at the Bay of Fundy in the Gulf of Maine.

In aeons past, the gravitational impact of the Moon would have been awesome, due to its proximity to Earth. A billion years ago, the tighter orbit of the Moon took fewer than twenty days, with eclipses frequent and dramatic. On low coastlands the marine ingress would have been extensive, creating the intermediate conditions for our evolutionary beginnings. Upper shore creatures gradually developed lungs for the interval between tides, some adapting to permanent habitat on land. The tides are gradually weakening as the Moon, currently at an average distance of 238,757 miles, is pulled outwards under centrifugal force. Earth rotates faster than the Moon revolves, but the spinning motion is slowing, and in fifty billion years terrestrial day and lunar month will be equal.

For early civilisations, the Moon was the index of time, and the derivation of 'month' is obvious. The lunar calendar is maintained in the semitic religions of Judaism and Islam, and the Christian festival of Easter has lunar-solar timing, occurring on the first Sunday after the full moon following vernal equinox (when the Sun crosses the equator in mid-spring, making day and night equal). The great psychoanalyst Carl Gustav Jung (1875–1961), who regarded myth as inherent to human thought, saw in the Moon a projection of the collective unconscious, its perpetual lunar cycles

---

1   The gravitational force of the Sun is 175 times larger than that of the Moon, but our satellite has the dominant tidal force because tides are caused by the difference in gravity field across Earth. The diameter of Earth is a tiny fraction of the distance to the Sun, but the Moon is so close that it causes twice as much change in the terrestrial gravity field. The difference in tidal force follows Newton's inverse square law.

of birth, growth, decay, death and rebirth representing both profane human mortality and the sacred eternity of the heavens. Ideas of reincarnation were inspired by the transforming Moon. The Sumerians believed that their lunar goddess Nannu hung dead for three days and nights on a hook in the Great Below, until she was revived by the food of life, and rose again to the Great Above, collecting her veils and jewels of light on her way. As people feared the wrath of gods, the appearance of the slim curve of new moon was a cause for ritual celebration. Transcending cultures and centuries, the waxing moon has meant beginnings: marriage, conception, sowing; the waning moon culmination: harvesting, reflecting, mourning.

In an agrarian existence, life ran to a lunar schedule. 'Harvest moon' appears around autumn equinox on the northern hemisphere, when a succession of evenings are graced by a luxuriant disc, the traditional feast honouring its deliverance of nature's bounty. Lunar cultivation survives in isolated farming communities, and has been revived by New Age lifestylers. The earliest known lunar growing calendar was prepared by Hesiod in the eighth century BC. Systematic investigation of plant growth in relation to the Moon was begun by Francis Bacon in the sixteenth century, and more recent experiments give tentative support to the old belief that root crops grow best if planted when the Moon is waning, and exposed crops under a waxing moon. Until the revolution in France, felling of trees was permitted only under a waning moon, when the wood was supposed to be more dry and resistant to weevils. The connection with water would have been reinforced by the coincidence of dew and full moon (for which a rational explanation is the rapid radiation of heat from Earth on cloudless nights, when the Moon shines brightest). However, a scientific basis may yet be found in changes in soil moisture. In the 1970s biologist Frank A Brown reported a statistically significant correlation between water absorption of bean seeds and lunar phases, although other workers in the field have suspected bias in his results. Indisputable, however, is that some types of leaves and flowers open in the direction of the Moon.

The biodynamic movement of Austrian philosopher-clairvoyant Rudolf Steiner (1861–1925) promotes organic farming on the basis that all liquids are subject to aethereal cosmic forces, dominated by the zodiacal trajectory of the Moon, which in occult belief governs growth and change of form. In the 1920s Lilo Kolisko in Stuttgart reported higher growth in corn and other plants when planted just before full moon. A follower of Steiner, Kolisko initiated the study of capillary dynamolysis, whereby plant sap activity is related to the aspect of the Moon and planets, as described in her book The Moon and Plant Growth. In the 1950s Maria Thun conducted systematic research on crop yields related to the sidereal position of the Moon. Best results were obtained when root, leaf, flower and fruit cops were sown when the Moon occupied the constellations associated with earth, water, air and fire respectively. Her astrological gardening calendar has been published annually since 1962. As well as an expanding range of books on lunar planting, enthusiasts can purchase an electronic clock, introduced in 1976 by the Burpee seed company, showing the Moon phases for sowing. While mainstream scientists regard the influence as minor and of little predictive value, weather almanacs based on lunar cycles are supported by evidence of increased precipitation approaching new and full moon.

Without doubt, the Moon has a profound effect on some animals. As eloquently described by Rachel Carson in her trilogy on marine life in the 1950s, creatures of the seashore must respond to the high tides occurring at intervals of twelve-and-three-quarter hours, and the low tides between. Oysters and other shellfish depend on the tides for their existence, as it brings food they cannot otherwise pursue; there is a fine balance between being under-nourished or marooned on land. The body clock of some littoral organisms is a compromise between lunar and solar regulation; for example, the camouflage of the fiddler crab responds to both tides and daylight. Predators further up the food chain are inevitably affected by the lunar patterns of smaller organisms, such as wading birds. Some nocturnal insects fly lower at full moon, probably to reduce detection by bats and other predators.

In 1769 Spaniards venturing up the Pacific coast were told by Californian Indians that fish danced on the sand at full moon. That this was no primitive fantasy was demonstrated to the incredulous visitors. Carried on the crest of a wave, countless fishes emerged on the shore to engage in a momentary lunar ball with their partners. The eggs of the grunion are laid beyond the normal tide level, where they are simultaneously fertilised by gyrating males, the interval between spring tides allowing time for incubation in the warm sand. The fishlet remains in its membrane until it is liberated by the next high tide a fortnight later. Aristotle, founder of scientific enquiry, noted that sea urchins were larger and tastier at full moon, and in the 1920s English biologist H Munro Fox confirmed that the reproductive pattern of this mollusc follows the synodic lunar cycle.[2] The spawning of oysters peaks at spring tides, which closely follow new and full moon.

Lunar regulation is most colourfully displayed by the palolo worm of the south Pacific. This invertebrate burrows underwater in rocks and corals on the coasts of Fiji and Samoa, and surfaces twice each year, at the neap tides of last quarter in October and November. Swarms of the reproductive segments rise to the surface, and by the next day the proliferation of eggs and spermatozoa causes the blue ocean to become a resplendent pink. Such occasions are celebrated by the native people, and provide an annual feast for sharks and other fish (there are always leftovers from the

---

2   Fox HM (1923): 'Lunar periodicity in reproduction'. *Proceedings of the Royal Society of London*, 95: 523–550.

banquet, allowing successful breeding). As the palolo worm lives in coral rocks three to five metres below the surface, it seems unlikely that moonlight is the governing factor. Chronobiology, the study of physiological rhythms in living organisms, had presumed a predominantly exogenous timing of daily and monthly cycles, but today an almost entirely inbuilt regulation is accepted. Intrinsic timing was confirmed in marine organisms by continuation of rhythmicity beyond exposure to the ebb and flow of ocean tides. In an aquarium, the *Convoluta roscoffensis* worm of Brittany rises from sand twice daily, to the exact timing of the low tides in its natural setting.

However, chronobiologist Frank A Brown argued that the persistence of rhythmicity in controlled experiments did not disprove a photic cue, because organisms may have higher sensitivity to light at particular times of day, so that constant light maintains a single daily signal. Brown examined the influence of environmental forces other than light and tides by taking oysters from the coast of Connecticut to his laboratory a thousand miles away at Northwestern University at Evanston, Illinois. In this inland setting they were placed in pans of sea water with no external stimuli. Oysters normally open their shells at high tide, when the Moon rises overhead. Initially, the pattern adhered to the timing of their distant habitat, but after a fortnight the oysters responded to the zenith of the Moon in Illinois. Rather than following a fixed timing, the oysters had somehow adjusted to their change of location. Observing correlation between biological cycles and fluctuations in geomagnetism, Brown speculated that the rhythm of life is set by the magnetic field. Biologists have confirmed that some amphibians and migratory birds respond to fluctuations in geomagnetism, and as the Moon affects Earth's magnetic field, this would at least partially explain correlations observed between the activity of some animals and the lunar cycle. On reviewing the theory and evidence, Tsutomu Nishimura and Masanori Fukoshima of Kyoto University proposed 'that animals respond to the full moon because of change in geomagnetic fields, and that the the the sensitivity of animal magnetoreception increases at this time'.[3]

The Moon, therefore, has proven influence on the rhythms of wildlife at the intermediary of land and sea, but does it affect the four-legged beasts of forest and plain? Full moonlight would appear to provide an accessory to the carnivore. However, a research team at the Fundação Zoo-Botânica in Brazil, on attaching satellite geographical locators to the collars of maned wolves in a vast savannah nature reserve at Minas Gerais, found that these solitary nocturnal hunters covered nearly two kilometres less distance at full moon than at new moon. The authors concluded that as

---

3   Nishumara T, Fakushima M (2009): 'Why animals respond to the full moon: magnetic hypothesis'. *Bioscience Hypotheses*, 2: 399– 401.

rodents and other animals reduce their activity at full moon due to increased predator risk, the wolves conserved energy at this time.[4] The legend of the werewolf, according to Robert Eisler's scholarly account *Man into Wolf*, began when primitive humankind was forced to append meat to its hitherto herbivorous diet. Envying the prowess of the wolf, and perhaps to invoke its spirit, men of hunting groups dressed in furs and painted their faces with lupine markings. Man was no match for the ghostly agility of the wolf, and the veneration and awe of their hungry competitor may have inspired the myth of metamorphosis. While the wolf was coveted for its qualities, it also came to represent sinister forces of the night. As wolves tended to howl at full moon, a person acting strangely at this time might be suspected of conversion to werewolf. By the seventeenth century lycanthropy had been reframed as a form of madness, and cases are occasionally reported in the psychiatric journals today. Intriguingly, research has shown an increase in animal bites at full moon, including a study of human victims at an accident and emergency department of a British hospital.[5]

Regarding lunar influence on human beings, the modern scientific establishment (with some notable exceptions such as Carl Sagan) has tended to dismiss such ideas as a relic of folklore. It was very different in the past, when great thinkers such as Aristotle were convinced that people were affected by the phases of the Moon. As encyclopaedist of the arcane Fred Gettings explained, the etymology of the term 'influence' relates to the Moon and stars, the 'flowing into' implying aethereal spirit passing from macrocosm to microcosm. In its waxing and waning, the Moon was believed in ancient wisdom to regulate the energies of life, as described by Roman naturalist Pliny the Elder:[6]

> We may certainly conjecture that the Moon is not unjustly regarded as the star of our life. This it is that replenishes the Earth; when she approaches it, she fills all bodies, while, when she recedes, she empties them. From this cause it is that shell-fish increase with the increase of the Moon and that bloodless creatures especially feel breath at that time; even the blood of men grows and diminishes with the light of the Moon, and leaves and herbage also feel the same influence, since the lunar energy pervades all things.

In ancient Greece, lunar goddess Artemis was protector of pregnant women, a likely factor being that labour begins almost twice as frequently

4   Sábato MAL, de Melo LFB, Magni EMV, Young RJ, Coelho CM (2006): 'A note on the effect of the full moon on the activity of wild maned wolves, Chysocyon brachyurus'. *Behavioural Processes*, 73: 228–230.

5   Bhattacharjee C, Bradley P, Smith M, Scally AJ, Wilson BJ (2000): 'Do animals bite more during a full moon? Retrospective observational analysis'. *British Medical Journal*, 321: 1559–1560.

6   *Pliny (c77–79). Naturalis Historia.* Quoted by Jules Cashford in lecture to the Analytical Psychology Club, London, October 2004 (accessed 10 September 2010 at www.goddessreligion.pbworks.com).

at midnight as at noon. As well as its perceived role as midwife, the Moon has also been associated with fertility. Throughout the ages, menstruating women have been considered to be in harmony with the Moon. South American Indians believed that all human life was made from 'moon blood'. Charles Darwin in his *Descent of Man* (1871) suggested that the similar duration of menstrual and lunar periods was an artefact of distant stages in evolution, when the tides stamped their authority on all animal life: 'Man is subject, like other mammals, birds, and even insects, to that mysterious law, which causes certain normal processes, such as gestation, as well as the maturation and duration of various diseases, to follow lunar periods.'

There is an obvious flaw in the idea that the menses are regulated by the Moon. Confronting this common belief, astronomer George O Abell in his book *Science and the Paranormal* (1983), asked why lunar periodicity does not apply equally to other mammals: sheep have a cycle of sixteen to seventeen days, rats five days, and macaque monkeys twenty-five days. Indeed Abell noted that the human period is one-and-a-half days shorter than the lunar cycle, although this was accepting the popular but inexact duration of twenty-eight days. From a large data set, Walter and Abraham Menaker reported in the *American Journal of Obstetrics and Gynaecology* in 1959 that a high proportion of women's cycles do not merely approximate the synodic period, but match its length of twenty-nine-and-a-half days. Furthermore, on examining birth records over a nine-year period in New York hospitals, they found an average period of gestation in quarter-of-a-million births of exactly nine lunar months. Some evidence has been found for synchronicity of the beginning of menstruation with lunar phases, supporting the observation of the Aristotle that the effluence coincided with a waning moon. In a paper *Cosmic Influences on Physiological Phenomena* in 1898, one of the earliest scientific reports of human biological rhythms, Svante Arrhenius reported correlation of lunar and menstrual cycles, although this finding was neither replicated by Dunn, Jenkin and Gunn in 1937, nor by Pochobradsky in 1974.

The Menakers had also reported that more babies were born in the days after full moon, supporting the traditional belief in midwifery. However, from twenty years of data, Abell and Greenspan found no link between the Moon and motherhood. A recurring theme in this book is the conflicting science of lunar influence, exemplified by two maternity studies published in 1998. Mathematicians at Urbino University in Italy analysed the synodic distribution of 1,248 spontaneous deliveries, and found statistically significant clustering around full moon.[7] The other study at Long Island College Hospital in Brooklyn found no correlation, authors Joshi

---

7 Ghiandoni G, Secli R, Rocchi MBL, Ugolini G (1998): 'Does lunar position influence the time of delivery? A statistical analysis'. *European Journal of Obstetrics and Gynaecology and Reproductive Biology*, 77: 47– 50.

and colleagues concluding: 'Scientific analysis does not support the belief that the number of births increases as the full moon approaches, therefore it is a myth not reality'.[8] Scientific doctrine insists that a single negative finding refutes a hypothesis, but an ongoing accumulation of results both for and against a lunar effect suggests something amiss with the methodology.

Biologist Winnifred Cutler claimed that the independence between Moon and menses found by researchers was because they had not isolated women with cycles of circalunar duration. In 1980 she conducted a prospective double-blind study of 312 students at the University of Pennsylvania. Users of oral contraceptives were excluded, and only one student per dormitory was enrolled, thus avoiding the confounding effect of converging tendencies in co-resident women. A disproportionate number of the 68 women with cycles of around twenty-nine-and-a-half days ovulated in the dark phases of the moon (the half-cycle centred on new moon). Cutler continued her research on the link between the Moon and female rhythms, and in 1986 she founded the Athena Institute for Women's Wellness Research in Philadelphia, declaring on its website: 'My research has consistently focused on what behaviour a woman can engage in to increase her power, well-being, vitality and sexual pleasure'.

The most intriguing conjecture on the Moon, and the focus of this book, is in its powers on the mind. The mystical but universal lunar link to madness in the ancient world was rationalised by Aristotle and Galen as the result of fluid regulation, insanity having a physiological basis in excessive moisture on the brain. Whatever the mechanism, the idea has survived beyond through monotheism and the Age of Reason into modern society, although it cannot be found in the textbooks of biology, or in the manuals of mental health professions. The psychiatric profession (only two hundred years old) began in asylums for 'lunatics', but such terminology was a cultural artefact institutionalised by eighteenth-century lawyers, and soon abandoned by doctors as a diagnostic label. For the Moon to inflict symptoms of mental illness violates the assumptions of modern clinical psychiatry, a discipline that has distanced itself from lay conceptualisations of mental disorder. Yet belief in lunar influence persists in mental health nursing—the profession with the most enduring contact with patients.

Anecdotal accounts of a lunar effect by nurses may be casually dismissed as the unscientific thinking of a relatively less educated body of workers. As in science generally, the esotericism of psychiatry has a conservative tendency, and the phenomenon described by sociologists as knowledge closure can suppress observations from further down the

8   Joshi R, Bharadwaj A, Gallousis S, Matthews R (1998): 'Labor ward workload waxes and wanes with the lunar cycle, myth or reality?' *Primary Care Update for Ob/Gyns*, 5: 184.

pecking order. 'Doctor knows best' was recently confronted by a cat in a Rhode Island nursing home.[9] Care workers were convinced that Oscar, an unremarkable tabby, had a sixth sense in predicting deaths. He would snuggle beside residents in their last hours of life, and often imminent deaths would not otherwise have been anticipated by staff. The animal was possibly able to detect decaying cells, a similar phenomenon having been observed with dogs. The author, professor of geriatric medicine David Dosa, humbly acknowledged that he was the last to accept the validity of this feline premonition, but without someone of his status taking it seriously, Oscar would have remained unknown beyond his pastel-shaded domain. If persuasive evidence of lunar influence on the mind arises, mental hospital nurses across the world would deserve credit — and perhaps an apology!

In recent decades, the lunar hypothesis has been subjected to a flurry of systematic investigation, with equivocal findings. One might presume that proving or disproving a lunar effect would be straightforward, but as we shall see, it is rather more complicated than that.

Nonetheless, some writers have seen enough in the data to conclude lunar influence on behaviour. In his book *How the Moon Affects You*, Miami psychiatrist Arnold Lieber presented results of his research on lunar correlation with aggression, asserting that the human being is 'a symphony of rhythms', in tune with cosmic forces not currently understood: With its circular reasoning and selective reporting, his treatise is unlikely to sway the sceptic; here is unquestioning belief in 'something out there'. By contrast, mainstream scientific opinion is often coloured by extreme scepticism. In an otherwise excellent book on the Moon, BBC science correspondent David Whitehouse dismissed outright the idea of lunar influence on behaviour. 'Be warned', he wrote, 'some readers will not like what I am about to say in this chapter'. His review showed bias similar to that found in Lieber's book. Rather like Richard Dawkins in his bestselling polemic *The God Delusion*, which caricatures Christianity by the fundamentalist preachers of the Bible Belt, Whitehouse selected anecdotal accounts of no scientific validity, then criticised these for being anecdotal. He stated that 'suicides show no lunar effect' as if accepted fact, ignoring the evidence to the contrary. This is not refined meta-analysis, but unmerited absolutism.

The issue takes us to the heart of what is science. We like to think that in our trajectory of progress we have replaced myth and magic with logic and reason. Forty years ago, the BBC produced two monumental documentaries: Kenneth Clark's *Civilisation*, and *The Ascent of Man*, presented

9   Dosa D (2007): *Making Rounds with Oscar: The Extraordinary Gift of an Ordinary Cat.* New York: Hyperion.

by J Bronowski.[10] While the former focused on artistic and cultural development, the latter charted the advance of science. Both series had profound messages on intellectual endeavour. According to philosopher and socialist Bertrand Russell, the criterion of an enlightened society is foresight, but Clark counselled against such one-way vision: 'Civilised man must feel that he belongs somewhere in space and time; that he consciously looks forward and looks back'.[11] Science and technology appear to advance as a linear process of accretion, whereby we build on the discoveries and learn from the errors of the past. Arthur Koestler began his admirable history of cosmology *The Sleepwalkers* by stating: 'We can add to our knowledge, but we cannot substract from it'. However, in the 1960s philosopher of science Thomas Kuhn described a revolutionary process of fits and starts, whereby a prevailing schema is torn apart by a new discovery or idea. Einstein's theory of relativity, for example, completely changed the rules of engagement in physics. Knowledge does not equate to the sum of concrete facts, but is a complex of subjectively demarcated constructs. We have made tremendous progress in understanding our place in the cosmos, but in the great maze of reality, surprises are always lurking around the corner. In his documentary, Bronowski emphasised the fundamental quality of the scientist: a doubting mind. It is in that spirit that we should consider the legendary link between the Moon and madness.

10   Bronowski J (1977): *The Ascent of Man*. London: Book Club Associates.
11   Clark K (1969/1999): *Civilisation: A Personal View*. London: Folio Society, p23.

One

Nearest heaven

From Chaos emerged Gaia, Mother Earth, and progenitress of the cosmos. With her son Ouranos, who embodied the sky and heavens, they created night and day, and the first generation of Titans. For imprisoning the Hundred-Handed and Cyclopes in the body of Gaia, Ouranos was castrated by Kronos, his eldest son. Kronos ruled in the Golden Age, before being overthrown by his sons Zeus, Pluto and Poseidon. After the Titans had devoured his son Zagreus, Zeus took revenge by striking them down with his thunderbolts. Banishing Kronos and the other Titans to the Underworld. Zeus became immortal, and governed the universe from the summit of Mount Olympus, leaving his brother Poseidon as master of the seas and Hades as ruler of the Underworld. As punishment for helping Kronos, Atlas was forced to carry Earth on his back. Zeus created moral order, and instructed Prometheus and Epimetheus to create mankind. Such was the beginning according to the Greeks, a dramatic cosmogeny as compelling in its time as the Big Bang theory of today.

In deference to the incredible forces of nature, ancient civilisations produced a myriad of fantasy, from which religion evolved. As illuminated by early twentieth-century sociologist Claude Lévi-Strauss, all mythologies had common themes of kinship, status and justice, suggesting inherent structural patterns in human development. From the Maya to the Chinese, Earth was posited as the centre of the universe. This flat expanse, with its uncharted nether regions, was bounded by a vast oceanic ring; at some faraway mysterium the seas ended and the unfathomable heavens began. With their anthropocentric star lore, early societies appointed priests, men or women considered to have special powers of interpretation and foresight, who could relate celestial patterns and events to terrestrial phenomena. Believing that they had little control on their destiny, people deferred to supernatural powers. An essential role of the priest was to keep the community on the right side of the easily offended gods; ritual sacrifices were performed to avoid their terrifying wrath.

The Sun and the Moon, as the most prominent celestial bodies, were venerated. Seasonal fluctuations in the terrestrial environment were found to correlate with celestial patterns and were consequently attributed to divine government. In Egypt and Mesopotamia, the two cradles of western civilisation, livelihood depended on the annual flooding of rivers. As deliverer of feast or famine, the Nile was considered by the ancient Egyptians to be under the power of the Memphite god Osiris, while the Sun god Ra provided light and warmth for crops. It was believed that Ra, after setting in the west, was rowed by Osiris across an underground sea so that he could rise again in the east. The Moon too made a daily watery transit, as in the human–piscine Syrian lunar goddess Atargartis – the original mermaid – who represented the dark and its potentially dangerous passions.

Contributing to its mythological powers, the Moon made the least disciplined trajectory against the astral surround, and was alone in changing form; more than any other celestial body, it was held in awe. In early mythology, Moon and Sun were both regarded as male. Patriarchal hegemony was instilled by the Egyptians who incarnated Ra in the Pharaohs, while moon god Thoth was the deputy chief, and wise scribe of the heavens. By his nocturnal illumination, Thoth kept demons at bay, and prevented any attempt to overthrow Ra. The Mesopotamian moon god Sin, honoured by a temple in Babylon, was the most powerful of the astral trinity, alongside Ishtar (Venus) and Shamash (the Sun). Once the supremacy of the Sun was appreciated, with the Moon borrowing light from its more distant benefactor, a male–female dualism was established. Thoth was feminised in the form of his mistress Seshat, goddess of writing. The Moon remained a powerful figure, but its changing form contrasted with the eternal perfection of the Sun. In what would now be considered an expression of misogyny, the Sun was regarded as inherently male and rational, the Moon female and temperamental. Terrible powers of vengeance were exacted by the wantonly violent Anat, moon goddess of the Phoenicians, and by Kali Ma, the respective Hindu deity.

The Greeks had three goddesses associated with the Moon and its cycles. The lunar connection of Artemis, goddess of chastity and hunting, arose around the same time that her twin Apollo was linked to the Sun. The most beautiful Olympian deity, Artemis was welcomed as the waxing moon. She made the divine bond between women and nature, and was protector of the pregnant, although she could also inflict still-births and maternal death. The glowing full moon was represented by Selene (in Greek, *selas* meant light). Selene, who drove the moon chariot, was the sister of Helios (the Sun) and Eos (dawn), but was later considered to be daughter of Helios, probably once the Moon was relegated in status. Finally, there was Hecate. Honoured by Zeus, Hecate was a mysterious triple goddess who was simultaneously powerful in Earth, the Heavens and the Underworld. Goddess of childbirth, she also brought darkness as the waning moon, and became associated with necromancy, sorcery and witchcraft (as celebrated at Hallowe'en). The Greeks saw the Moon as the gateway to the heavens, where souls were purified before passing on. As recorded by the Roman compiler Plutarch (AD 46–120), the large plain of the Elysian Fields was believed to be the place through which souls passed after death. Another sacred area was the Shrine of Hecate, one of the largest hollows on the lunar surface.

Although the founders of rational enquiry, the Greeks were deeply immersed in myth. Their gods, who dominated the lives of philosopher and fisherman alike, were honoured through rituals of chastity, solitude, fasting and pilgrimage. In his *Theogeny*, Hesiod produced a genealogy of the Greek pantheon. As in other ancient civilisations, their mythology was of multiple sources, a blend of early animistic deities and Dorian sky gods. People moving from the hinterlands to city states brought with them local myths, as embellished by the blind poet Homer in the chronicles *Iliad* and *Odyssey*. Myth, religion and actual events were entwined in Homer's verse, which has been described as an Aegean Bible. The Moon and stars, as the embodiment of the gods, presented moral order. The legendary interpretation of the wondrous spectacle of the Milky Way as the spilt breast milk of Hera did not simply result from scientific ignorance. For the Greeks there was no contradiction between *logos* and *mythos*. While the physical world could be described rationally, meaning in life was conferred through a rich tapestry of symbolic drama. The cycle of seasons, for example, was explained by the story of Persephone, the beautiful daughter of Demeter, goddess of agriculture. Hades abducted Persephone, but eventually Demeter found her, and it was agreed that Persephone could spend half of the year in the upper world, and the other half as queen of the Underworld. Each spring Persephone reappeared, bringing longer and warmer days. As mythologist Paul Veyne explained:

> Myth is truthful, but figuratively so. It is not historical truth mixed with lies; it is a high philosophical teaching that is entirely true, on the condition that, instead of taking it literally, one sees in it an allegory.[1]

In the light of advances in logic and natural philosophy, the Olympian deity was frequently revised, and in the fourth century BC Aristotle could confidently assert that Man was ruled less by gods than by himself. Nonetheless, Heroic myth flourished in the Hellenistic age, as embodied in the all-conquering Alexander the Great. The pantheon was adopted by the Romans. Jupiter was the direct equivalent of Zeus, and lunar deity Artemis appeared in the guise of Diana, whose cult was centred at Ephesus.

1   Veyne P (1988): *Did the Greeks Believe in their Myths? An Essay on the Constitutive Imagination* (translated P. Wissing). Chicago: University of Chicago Press, p. 62.

The two faces of Janus maintained the traditional dualism of Sun and Moon: the former conveying intelligence, rationale and industry; the latter the source of impulsive behaviour and madness. The Romans lacked the enquiring mind of the Greeks, and the gods had a long twilight before the ascendancy of the Christian creed.

For all the cumulative knowledge of Aegean scholars and their Egyptian and Babylonian predecessors, the story of the demystification of the Moon and stars is no linear passage of human enlightenment. Indeed, if Jung is to be believed, mysticism may be with us in perpetuity. Yet humankind has undoubtedly made great strides in understanding its place in the universe. Astronomy, the first body of knowledge meriting the modern label of 'science', was the beginning of this journey.

Calendar and zodiac

Chronological awareness was essential to human organisation, and time was set by the heavens. The most obvious unit was the day, marked by the diurnal setting and rising of the Sun. From the regular cycles of the Moon, the period of a month was established, depicted in Egyptian hieroglyphic symbols as a crescent. Etchings on Stone Age bones apparently depict the days of a lunar month, as does a curved series painted around 15000 BC in the Caves of Lascaux in Dordogne. Priests would announce the beginning of each month to their rulers, timed either by first sighting of new moon, or (if obscured by cloudy skies) the number of days elapsed since its last appearance. The path of the Sun around Earth in relation to the astral surround was termed the 'ecliptic' because the proximate trajectory of the Moon caused the frequent occurrence of lunar and solar eclipses. Priests embellished their reputation by learning to predict these events. Interpreted as divine disapproval, an eclipse was a convenient time to raise taxes.

The problem with the Moon was that no multiple of months matched exactly the annual progression. For an agrarian livelihood, the weather was a rough guide to the change of seasons, but costly mistakes such as sowing too early could cause famine. The stars provided the metric for mastering the concept of time, as priest–astronomers deciphered the period of approximately twelve months that the Sun took to reappear in the same position on the stellar backdrop. The vernal equinox was determined as the beginning of the solar year. As we now appreciate, the seasons result from the tilting of Earth as it revolves around the Sun, but for the ancients it sufficed to observe the progression of sunrise on the horizon. The spring equinox is when the Sun crosses a north–south line. Determining the precise length of the year was a complicated endeavour, which entailed patient charting of the stars at sunrise and sunset, and measurement of the Sun's shadow. The Inca used fixed points to follow the Sun on its ascent and descent from the meridian, while the solstitial and equinoctal festivities of pagan societies were marked by calendrical structures such as the Megalithic monument of Stonehenge. The calendar was not the ready-reckoner of today, but shrouded in esoteric mystique.

Advances in chronological awareness highlighted an awkward discrepancy between lunar and solar time, shattering notions of numerical perfection. Early civilisations had determined the year as a period of 360 days, but this was longer than twelve lunar months, and too short for the revolution of the Sun. The Egyptians, by indexing on a specific star, found that the Sun took 365 days to complete its revolution. There was practical benefit in this observation. Sirius, the brightest star, appeared on the dusk horizon at the end of each summer, and this heralded the great flooding of the Nile. The natural cause of the swell was heavy rainfall on the Abyssinian heights, but in the legendary interpretation this was goddess Sopdet weeping. On receding the river left swaths of rich mud on either side, and with their pragmatic bent, the Egyptians applied basic laws of geometry (literally, the measurement of land) in redrawing boundaries. The Great Pyramid in Gizeh, built around 2900 BC, had ventilation shafts positioned so that Sirius shone on the preserved head of the Pharaoh, and the imminent flood was announced. As the people relied on lunar months for managing their affairs, the authorities allowed a dual system, retaining the venerable 360 days for the civil calendar alongside the sidereal year marked by the heliacal rising of Sirius. The three seasons, each of four months, were *akhet* (inundation), *peret* (growth) and *shemu* (harvest). The Egyptians conferred on the High Priest of Heliopolis the title 'Observer of the Secrets of the Heavens', and on his direction the dates of festivals were shifted to reconcile the two calendars. To the 360-day year, five feast days were added to make up the shortfall. Eventually it became evident that the year lasted for a quarter of a day longer than 365, and over centuries this was enough for significant slippage.

The embryonic astronomy of the Egyptians almost certainly tapped into wisdom from further afield. The Sumerians, from the mountainous north-east of Mesopotamia, settled in the 'fertile crescent' between the rivers of the Tigris and Euphrates, and they were keen stargazers, recording their intricate observations in cuneiform symbols on clay tablets. To keep track with the Moon, the Sumerian year had twelve months of alternating length of twenty-nine or thirty days, producing a year of 354 days. This being too short, an additional month was added to the end of the year on an ad hoc basis. The Saros cycle of almost nineteen years in which most patterns of the Moon recur, determined in the fifth century BC by Greek astronomer Meton, was probably discovered independently by the Babylonians, whose intercalation was set at a frequency of three times in eight years. The thirteenth month was considered an unpropitious time for business and family affairs, and explains superstitious notions about the number 13. The Sumerians established the sexagesimal periods of minutes and seconds, and in their nominal year of 360 days, each day represented one degree of the heavenly dome. Here originated the 360-degree circle instilled by Greek mathematicians.

Around 2500 BC the Sumerians were assimilated by the Semitic tribes who overran Mesopotamia. Their Babylonian heirs produced timetables of celestial motions, and differentiated the planets from the other heavenly bodies. While the fixed stars retained the same relative positions, in what became known as the firmament, the seven planets, which included the Sun and Moon, wandered across a narrow belt, termed the zodiac. The Babylonian term for planets was *bibbu* (literally, wild goats). Believing that their fate was fixed by the heavens, the Babylonians embodied their chief gods and goddesses in the planets. The city god of Babylon and ultimate authority was Marduk (Jupiter), to whom the Tower of Babel was dedicated. As the brilliant light and capricious motion of Venus, Ishtar was third in the hierarchy of planets, behind the Sun (Shamash) and Moon (Sin). She was goddess of love, while red Nergal (Mars) was god of war. Unhurried Ninurta (Saturn) was revered as god of old age, while Nabu (Mercury) was the rapid messenger of the planets. The seven days of the week took the names of the planets, known today in their Roman adaptations. The derivation of Sunday, Monday and Saturday is clear, and while our other days are named from Norse mythology (Tiu, Woden, Thor and Freya), the planetary origin is retained in the French form.

Table 1.1 The week in planets

Planet	Day	Day (in French)
Sun	Sunday	*Dimanche*
Moon	Monday	*Lundi*
Mars	Tuesday	*Mardi*
Mercury	Wednesday	*Mercredi*
Jupiter	Thursday	*Jeudi*
Venus	Friday	*Vendredi*
Saturn	Saturday	*Samedi*

Alongside theological interpretations of the stars and planets, anthropocentrism was elaborated in astrology, an occult system with independent origins in early Mayan civilisation, in China, and in Mesopotamia. For millennia groups of stars had been imaginatively construed as two-dimensional figures of animals, people or implements, from which meanings were inferred. Astrology developed as a framework of celestial influence based loosely on the constellations and their mythological powers. Early Babylonian astrology was based on a lunar zodiac marked by eighteen constellations. The circle of twelve signs was devised by the Chaldeans, from the head of the Persian Gulf, whose warlike leader Nebuchadnezzar II (604–561 BC) ruled Mesopotamia and built the great city of Babylon with its Hanging Gardens. After the Persian conquest in 539 BC, the work of the renowned Chaldean astronomers continued. Demarcating the zodiac into equal arcs of thirty degrees on the ecliptic, the Chaldeans produced a comprehensive model to predict character, events and destiny.[2]

Although initially disparaged by the Greeks, astrology became popular following the imperial exploits of Alexander the Great. Retaining the Chaldean symbols, Hellenistic astrologers developed the system into a convoluted clock dial, with the constellations as twelve points and planets

2   The zodiac was also related to the constellations, from which the signs and symbols were taken. The malevolence of number thirteen appeared in the sidereal demarcation, as the twelve asterisms did not complete the zodiacal band. A thirteenth constellation was represented as serpent bearer Ophiucus. It was discarded by the Greeks due to the significance of number twelve, as expressed in the decahedron, one of the five perfect solids of geometry. Note however that the true zodiac is simply an equal division of the ecliptic. As explained in scholarly texts on astrology, the tropical sign Aries, for example, bears no relation to the constellation of that name in location or extent.

as seven hands. Whereas in other cultures the horoscope was the preserve of the ruling class, the Greeks made it accessible to all; prominence was given to natal astrology, whereby influence depended on which planet occupied the particular constellation on the day of birth. As the significator of personality, the Moon was a potent astrological body, traversing the zodiac faster than any other sphere, with full moon appearing in a different sign each month (always opposite the Sun on the zodiac); two people born a few days apart could have different disposition due to the changing lunar position. Relating to the imaginative, reflective aspects of the personality, a prominent Moon in the chart indicated a sensitive, impressionable nature; if adversely positioned, it gave rise to a withdrawn, morbid character, prone to misfortune.

Harmony of spheres

To the Greeks, the great sea that encircled land was represented by the god Oceanus, son of Gaia and Ouranos. Its far reaches were considered unnavigable; 'Here be dragons', warned the margins of nautical charts. An overzealous explorer, if not devoured by the monstrous serpents inhabiting its far reaches, would eventually plunge into the great abyss. More adventurous were the Phoenician merchants from the eastern edge of the Mediterranean, whose maritime excursions took them to India via the Red Sea, and through the Pillars of Hercules into the ocean that was believed to ultimately meet the sky. In their sturdy cedarwood galleys they reached the Atlantic island of Britain, where they traded for Cornish tin. The Phoenicians left no record of their voyages, but according to Herodotus, around 600 BC they circumnavigated Africa. In the absence of their guiding light, the Pole Star, which disappears below the horizon in the southern hemisphere, their entire journey would have straddled the coast.

Contrasting with the Egyptians, early Greek scholars had little interest in the humble task of observation; they were concerned with metaphysics, pursuing the laws of nature through the faculty of reason. Their universe was a physical and moral unity, essentially of simple constitution. The first great leap of cosmological imagination was made in the sixth century BC by Thales of Miletus (c627–c545 BC), a Greek colony in Asia Minor. Inspired by the mathematics and astronomy learned from his travels to Babylon and Egypt, Thales was a practical thinker who eschewed star lore and other popular myths, and he avoided reference to deity in explaining the physical world. He proposed water as the primordial substance of the universe, and depicted Earth as a raft floating on sea, the land mass resulting from a gradual silting process, just as a river forms a delta. Earthquakes were not acts of divine retribution but the result of turbulence in the waters below. By his accurate prediction of a total eclipse of the Sun on 28 May 585 BC, Thales demonstrated the possibility of deciphering the underlying orderliness of the heavens.

On his visits to Egypt, Thales would have noticed that the Ursula Major constellation, despite Homer's verse stating that this great beast never bathed in Oceanus, dipped below the desert horizon for a short time each night. Taking this as evidence that Earth could not be a flat square, his pupil Anaximander (c610–c547 BC) postulated a cylindrical column floating in space, equidistant from all other cosmic bodies. Consequently, the ocean was not a moat separating us from the heavens, but a feature of Earth itself. The stars were pin-holes in a black screen, with the Sun a larger aperture to the great inferno behind. This dramatic conceptualisation was too radical for Anaximander's contemporaries, but it was an important development. Whereas the Chinese, Egyptians and Mesopotamians had interpreted celestial motions as prognostic signs, Greek scholars presented the universe in entirely mechanical terms.

The quest to explain the perfection of the heavens was taken forward by an Ionian sage of the sixth century BC. The term *philosophos* meant lover of wisdom, and this was epitomised by mathematician and mystic Pythagoras of Samos (c570–c470 BC). He first used the term 'cosmos' to mean the order of the universe, and sought the hidden syntax in numerology. Following the death of the despot Polycratos, who had shown him favour, Pythagoras left Samos and in 531 BC established a religious academy at Kroton in the Greek colony of Magna Graecia, the southern tip of Italy. Immersed in Orphic mystery, Pythagoras and his reverent brotherhood propagated the idea of reincarnation, and pursued the secrets of eternity by attempting to synthesise the parallel worlds of nature and spirit. Music was the key. Pythagoras found that by stretching cords of varying length to the same tension, different sounds were emitted, and that similar ratios produced notes on a common scale. Musical instruments thus became one of the first practical applications of the precise measurement of natural phenomena. The human body was analogised to the tone and balances of the lyre, and the mathematical order of supposed interstellar distances suggested to Pythagoras a harmonic universe. The acoustic perfection of the macrocosm could not be heard by most people because their souls were out of harmony — until they died.

Pythagoras did not, as is commonly believed, introduce the term 'music of the spheres', as the distant stars were not conceptualised as rotund until the time of Eudoxus centuries later. However, appreciation of the Earth itself as an orb was a great intellectual step for mankind. Clues had been provided by mariners, whose voyages to northern latitudes brought a changing panorama of stars and longer summer days; another hint of curvature was in the masts of departing ships disappearing last from view. Pythagoras noticed that the shadow of Earth during a lunar eclipse was curved. The first known mention of Earth as a globe was by Parmenides of Elea in the fifth century BC, and this led to baffling contemplation on a lower hemisphere. Philolaus of Kroton (c470–390 BC), who brought Pythagorean mathematics and astronomy to the attention of Aristotle and Plato, was reputedly first to describe Earth as a moving body—not spinning, but with a daily revolution in space. Philolaus thought that Earth, planets and stars revolved around *antichton* (counter-Earth), which always faced the uninhabited side of Earth, just as the Moon shows only one side to us.

The Moon loomed large in ancient Greek thought. Anaximander is credited with explaining moonlight as solar reflection, and this led to speculation about lunar life forms. Pythagoras imagined great plants and beasts, nourished by long periods of unbroken sunlight. Anaxagoras (c500–428 BC) of Athens, knowing that solar eclipses occurred at new moon, took secularisation too far by claiming that both Sun and Moon were mere matter. For this impiety he was imprisoned, showing that intellectual freedom had its limits in a culture of moral truth. In 413 BC, moon lore determined the outcome of a major event in Greek military fortunes, as told by historian Thucycdides. At the Battle of Syracuse, General Nicias had decided to retreat, but as the Athenians were about to set sail, there was a lunar eclipse. Perceiving a bad omen, the departure was postponed. This proved a fatal error, as the battalion was destroyed and Nicias stoned to death.

Geometry defied

Scholars enthused by Pythagorean harmony were unable to provide a satisfactory account of the visible universe. The problem was the erratic motions of the planets, particularly the Moon, but also Mercury and Venus, which would inexplicably race ahead of the Sun, slow down and reverse in their course. This was not permissible in a system of planets suspended on transparent spheres. As the chimes of the musical universe faded, natural philosophy shifted towards materialism. In the fifth century BC, Empedocles of Acragas (c492–440 BC) introduced the classic four elements of earth, water, air and fire; these produced the qualities dry, moist, cold and hot respectively. Then came the atom theory of

Democritus (c460BC–370 BC), and musings on the microcosm-macrocosm. Among the big questions for philosophers were, 'What is real, and what is permanent?' In contrast to the constant flux ontology of Heraclitus of Pontus (?–c480 BC), Parmenides (c515 BC–?), the most prominent scholar of the Eleatic school, insisted on an unchanging reality. The latter reached its pinnacle in the dualism of Plato (427–347 BC), whereby visible phenomena are an imperfect version of the eternal form, which can only be elicited through reason.

Inspired by the long-dead Pythagoras, Plato posited reality in an underlying mathematical perfection. He asserted: 'We shall approach astronomy, as we do geometry, by way of problems, and ignore what is in the sky'.[3] The Academy he founded in 387 BC in Athens bore the inscription 'A Credit in Geometry is Required'. Plato receives bad press from historians of science for his disdain for empirical enquiry, but his contribution to astronomy was important. He demanded a rational model of uniform celestial motion, adhering to two fundamental principles: the shape of the world must be a perfect sphere; and all motion must be in perfect circles at uniform speed. Disciples of Plato rose to his challenge, and on the assumption that circular perfection was inherent to nature, attempted to construct a homogenous system.

First to respond was mathematical genius Eudoxus (c390–c340 BC) of Cnidus, who had studied for a year with the priests at Heliopolis, and whose geometry probably influenced Euclid. To explain the inconsistent motions of the planets, Eudoxus and his follower Calippus created a system of thirty-four geocentric spheres, with each planet fixed to a set of spheres on different axes. Both Sun and Moon had three cycles, and the other planets four each, circulating a stationary Earth. This original mathematical model of the cosmos set the tone of astronomy for the next two thousand years. Yet the flaws were obvious. Although the system equated roughly to the visible motions, it did not take account of the varying brightness of planets, particularly Venus, Mars and the Moon, which suggested fluctuating distance from Earth. To the frustration of Greek astronomers, the planets defied geometric discipline.

Heraclides of Pontus (c388–c315 BC), another pupil of Plato, was determined to show that the retrograde motion of Mars was not random, but a predictable feature of its revolution. In his novel theory, the planets revolved not as a purely circular motion, but turned in loops. As Mercury and Venus were more difficult to accommodate, Heraclides speculated that these errant planets were satellites of the Sun, turning on epicycles on the larger circumference of the solar orbit of Earth. Here was recognition of the celestial bodies not being solely in the dominion of Earth, and the first step towards heliocentrism. Heraclides also asserted that Earth

3   Plato (1955): *The Republic*. Harmondsworth: Penguin.

rotated on its axis, thus explaining why the stars moved together (a conclusion first drawn in the fourth century BC by Nicetas of Syracuse), but this was generally rejected: the clouds would be limited to one direction, and the extreme spinning motion would throw off all traces of life.

Plato's mathematical cosmos was laden with creation mythology as the expression of divine perfection, but by contrast his pupil Aristotle (384–322 BC) devised a logical structure for the universe. Son of a physician in Macedonia, Aristotle studied for twenty years at the Academy, but rarely mentioned Plato in his works. He founded the Lyceum as a centre of empirical enquiry, contrasting with the almost anti-scientific teaching of the Academy. Theory was to be generated from evidence, with concrete facts the building blocks of knowledge. Whereas Plato saw change as degeneration from ideal form, Aristotle considered states as actual and potential, with nature guiding a final purpose. This teleology required an 'unmoved mover', which was the ultimate being. Crucial to his contribution to cosmology was the distinction he made between mathematics and mechanics: the former was limited to abstraction, while the latter described material process.

An enduring doctrine of Aristotlean cosmology was the spatial division of the universe into the natural and spiritual, bridging the philosophical dualism of Heraclitean 'becoming' (one cannot step into the same river twice) and Parmenidan 'being'. Change occurred only in the sublunar domain, where there was birth and death, and ongoing transformation between the four elements: earth and water, which had descending nature (gravity); and the ascending air and fire (levity). In the words of Arthur Koestler, the Aristotlean status of the Earth and the Moon was 'the disreputable slum district of the Universe'.[4] From the Moon outwards was incorruptible perfection, where the natural motion was eternal cycle. The stars were believed to consist of a fifth aethereal element, the invisible quintessence. Building on the geometrical system of Eudoxus, Aristotle's Earth was enclosed, like the skins of an onion, by nine concentric spheres, the innermost consisting of the elements water, air and fire, then came the crystalline spheres of the Moon, Sun and planets, and finally the 'stellatum'. He introduced a mechanical separation of the cycles, with intermediate spheres turning in the opposite direction of the planets, preventing one planetary orbit from interfering with another. Aristotle's addition of twenty-one spheres produced a total of fifty-five, but his contribution did more to complicate than explain the elusive planetary system.

From the third century BC onwards, astronomy was centred at Alexandria, the port metropolis founded by Alexander the Great. Dominated by

4   Koestler A (1964): *The Sleepwalkers: A History of Man's Changing Vision of the Universe.* Harmondsworth: Penguin, p59.

the Pharos lighthouse, one of the Seven Wonders of the World, this cosmopolitan city was at the heart of the Hellenistic empire and the seat of scientific scholarship, with a magnificent library containing thousands of scrolls on all branches of knowledge. One of its librarians was Eratosthenes (c285–194 BC) of Cyrene, who is most famous for calculating the circumference of Earth. Eratosthenes noticed that at midday of summer equinox, the Sun produced no shadow in the south of Egypt at Syene, being directly overhead, whereas in Alexandria a long shadow appeared. Following this observation, he had the distance between the two sites measured by men on foot. The distance being 252,000 *stadia*, he calculated a difference of 7 degrees, from which he estimated a circumference. His accuracy cannot be assessed precisely as the length of a *stade* is unkown, but he was probably within a few per cent of the correct figure of 24,880 miles.

While at Alexandria, Aristarchus (c310–230 BC) of Samos proposed a novel cosmology in which Earth lost its central status, joining the other planets in orbit around the Sun. The heliocentric thesis was reputedly first proposed by Pythagoras, probably based on the observed motions of the inner planets, but his works are lost. Sadly, so too is the key text of Aristarchus. However, his short treatise *On the Size and Distance of the Sun and Moon* survives, and this demonstrates his rigorous method. He estimated the diameter of the Moon, with only 8 per cent error. On observing the shadow of the Earth at lunar eclipse, Aristarchus concluded that the Sun must be far more distant than previously thought, and about ten times larger than Earth. Perhaps it was this observation that raised his doubts about an enormous Sun revolving around Earth.

We know of the heliocentric argument of Aristarchus through Archimedes (287–212 BC), the greatest mathematician and engineer of antiquity. For many years the Romans had been held at bay by military defences designed by Archimedes, but in 211 BC Syracuse was sacked, and the practical scholar was slain by a drunken soldier. The work of Archimedes remained highly influential, and the cogent argument of his book *Arenarius* was enough to put the Sun back in its subordinate place. For all their wisdom, the Greeks missed the signpost, and did not deviate from the thoroughfare of geocentrism. It was counter-intuitive for the Earth to move around the Sun; even with the underestimated distance, this would have required a miraculous speed of orbit. The model of Aristarchus, to be accepted, would have thrown the already convoluted knowledge of planetary motions into disarray. The failure of Greek scholarship was due not to religious intolerance but to their immersion in Platonic dogma and Aristotlean physics.

The wheeled universe

Around 250 BC, a creative solution to the planetary puzzle was offered by mathematician Apollonius of Perga. Applying conic sections to the problems of cosmic geometry, he described the variable motion of Mars as an eccentric orbit of varying distance from Earth. Although its distance from Earth was irregular, the planet swept equal areas of arc over time. The eccentric thesis, combined with the epicycles of Eudoxus, was pursued by Hipparchus (190–120 BC) of Rhodes, who pursued uniformity not through speculative theory, but by disciplined enquiry. Indeed, he is recognised as the originator of observational astronomy. Unlike his Greek predecessors, Hipparchus had access to the archives of Babylonian astronomers, and he built on their accurate records and methods of calculation. He tabulated the position and magnitude of over a thousand fixed stars, discovering a new star in the process. Around 150 BC he reported that the vernal equinox as observed by the Babylonians had changed, the position of the Sun having moved from the zone of Aries into Pisces, thus refuting the presumed permanence of the zodiac. This discovery of the precession of equinoxes, a cycle of 26,000 years, was crucial to later progress in astronomy. Hipparchus calculated that the stars shifted one degree from the terrestrial perspective every hundred years (this is now known to take seventy years).[5]

Hipparchus was also aware that longitude, necessary for the production of accurate maps, could be measured by the timing of lunar eclipses at multiple locations, although this work was not finished. By this time Alexandrian astronomers were using trigonometry to calculate planetary distances. At a solar eclipse in 129 BC, Hipparchus used the parallax of two reference points to determine the distance of the Moon from Earth. At Hellespont, on the eastern edge of the Greek mainland, the eclipse was total, while at Alexandria the Moon was a fifth of a solar diameter short of overlap. The difference amounted to 0.1 degree of the sky, and Hipparchus took the latitudes of the two points to estimate a distance averaging between 62 and 73 Earth radii—only slightly excessive. Like Aristarchus, Hipparchus suggested that the Sun and Moon were distant from Earth on a ratio of 20:1, much smaller than the actual ratio of 400:1.

5   There is no precise date, but the Age of Pisces is generally considered to have begun in the first or second century BC. As the retrograde motion of the vernal point covers 30 degrees of arc every 2,160 years, we must be in or approaching the Age of Aquarius. Christianity having coexisted with the Piscean period explains the piscine symbol of this religion.

Classic Greek philosophy was absent: here was the universe described with no attempt at meaning. Hipparchus was unable to complete the eccentric model started by Apollonius. To his disillusionment, the cycles of Mars and other planets were even more irregular than realised. This failure of centuries of Greek astronomy mirrored the demise of the Hellenistic empire, swept aside by the Romans. Was this the vengeance of the Olympic gods?

With its rational discourse on morals and nature, Greek culture had an enduring influence on the Roman world. Better known for their military superiority and administrative skill than scientific endeavour, the Romans made use of astronomy in eradicating the confusion of the lunisolar calendar. After consulting Alexandrian astronomer Sosigenes, in 46 BC Julius Caesar established a secular calendar, with a leap day every four years, an intercalation with an error of only eleven minutes.[6] Meanwhile, unfettered by its Latin rulers, Alexandria retained its intellectual lure. Here in the second century AD emerged a cosmology that worked not only in theory but in reality. Its author was Claudius Ptolemy (AD 85–165), the last great astronomer of the Alexandrian school.

Although Ptolemy rejected the Babylonian arithmetical methods used by Hipparchus, which he found lacked consistency and logic, he was intrigued by the eccentric and epicyclic thesis. With his Platonist bent, Ptolemy accepted that the objective of astronomy was to determine the consistent, circular motions of spheres in their diurnal revolution around Earth. In his thirteen-volume masterpiece *Mathematike Syntaxis* (translated by the Arabs as *Almagest*, meaning 'the greatest'), he described the Universe as a homogenous structure, with the planets revolving on epicycles at the end of imaginary spokes emanating from Earth. As Koestler described, the system operated like a giant ferris wheel. Each pod of the wheel revolved in its own cycle, but as the main wheel was continually turning, the motion was not seen as a circle but as a curvilinear trajectory. To improve accuracy, this behemoth with its total of forty cycles revolved on a point proximate to Earth. Ptolemy made concession to the precession of equinoxes described by Hipparchus by including a ninth sphere, which moved the fixed stars slowly backwards. For fourteen centuries the Ptolemaic system would be the uncontested truth.

---

6   An accumulating discrepancy of eleven minutes between calendar and solar year was long enough to become a theological problem, most noticeably with the moveable feast of Easter, which was occurring progressively earlier, the vernal equinox having regressed by ten days since the Council of Nicaea in 325. In 1582, following advice from astronomer Aloysius Lilius and Jesuit scholar Claivius, the current calendar was introduced by Pope Gregory XIII, which omits three of the extra days every four hundred years. In Britain the Gregorian calendar was instilled by Act of Parliament in 1752, and in Russia and other parts of eastern Europe the Julian calendar was not replaced until the early twentieth century.

Ptolemy maintained the sublunary and divine division of the universe, a Platonic dualism later instilled in Christian dogma. He also produced the leading text on astrology. While the Babylonian horoscope had filled a societal vacuum left by the decline of the Greek pantheon, Alexandrian scholars applied their geometric skill in refining planetary tables relating to the tropical zodiac. Astrology was thus blended with mythology and principles of natural philosophy, and was absorbed by Roman society. Emperor Tiberius took a keen interest in his horoscope, and fortune-telling became a lucrative enterprise on the streets of Rome. In his four-volume *Tetrabiblos*, described by Fred Gettings as 'a rationalised compendium of astrological lore',[7] Ptolemy defined the discipline as the probabilistic application of astronomy to terrestrial phenomena. He focused on the natural astrology of general celestial influence, rather than the judicial astrology often practised by unscrupulous fortune tellers. The Sun, Moon and planets were categorised by their heating, cooling, moistening and drying capacities, and by gender; the Moon, for example, was moist and thus female. As we shall see, belief in celestial influence on human welfare was soon to be restricted — not by advances in knowledge, but by religious doctrine.

Early medicine and lunar influence

The repertoire of the priest in early civilisation included the beginnings of medical practice. The power of gods was invoked to dispel the bad spirits deemed responsible for an affliction, and just as today a prescribed drug such as an antidepressant might sometimes be credited erroneously for a patient's self-remission, recipients of priestly medicine would have thanked the gods rather than the healing powers of their own bodies. Archaeological finds reveal that trephining of the skull was performed in many cultures, probably as a means of casting out bad spirits. Medicine and surgery were established as specialised occupations in China and Mesopotamia by 3000 BC, but the first known doctor was Imhotep in Egypt. Primarily an architect, Imhotep designed the Step Pyramid, and little is known of his therapeutic practice. However, such was his reputation that after his death he was immortalised as god of medicine. Papyri show that Egyptian physicians of the third millennium BC were using surgical implements, splints and a plethora of remedies prepared from animal and

7   Gettings F (1990): *The Arkana Dictionary of Astrology*. London: Penguin, p505.

plant extracts, but spells and incantations were also administered, guided by the wisdom of Thoth.

Greek medicine had spiritual authority in Apollo as god of health, and in the legendary healer Asklepius, who lived around 1250 BC, but was later deified. In myth, after saving too many people from death's door, Asklepius was struck by a thunderbolt from Zeus for interrupting the work of Hades. People sought divine remedy at Delphi, where Apollo had slain a serpent to allow safe habitation, and at the Asklepian temples of Epidaurus and throughout the Greek archipelago. Stone tablets record the curative results of incubation. A notable dissident to the supernatural interpretation of illness was Hippocrates (c460 BC–?), who observed that for all the reliance on amulets, incantations, herbs and oracles, worshipping of the gods seemed to make little difference in outbreaks of epidemic disease. Hippocrates asserted that medicine, as a craft, must be based on observation. The hundred volumes of the *Corpus Hippocraticum* lodged at the library of Alexandria, which were of multiple authorship, emphasised natural aetiology. Much influence was attributed to the climate and seasons, which governed the four fundamental qualities of hot, cold, dry and moist. In the treatise *On the Nature of Man*, the body was a vessel of four humours: blood, phlegm, yellow bile and black bile. Each person had one dominant humour, and a unique balance, requiring a detailed history to find and rectify the bodily upset. In the naïve physiology of the time, this model was supported by vomiting, the mucus of common colds, and non-traumatic nosebleeds, all of which suggested an excess of humour as the malady. The relationship of bodily fluids with the elements and physical qualities was later reinforced by Aristotlean natural philosophy.

Hippocratic medicine opposed mystical treatments, and the use of charms, often sold without scruple. Yet the Greek people had great faith in the cult of Asklepius, of which the most famous sanctuary was at Kos, birthplace of Hippocrates, where large numbers of pilgrims sought miraculous cure. Indeed, the Hippocratic Oath, a pledge taken by doctors to this day, referred to the ultimate authorities: 'I swear by Apollo the Physician, by Asklepius, by Hygiea, by Panacea, and by all the gods and goddesses.'[8]

Any condition of periodicity was likely to be associated with lunar cycles, as with the 'menses', a Latin term meaning a period determined by the Moon's course. Roman physicians applied the label *lunaticus* to people with recurring attacks of mental disturbance at full moon. Manifestations included not only aberrations of emotion and reason, but also convulsions, suggesting that the traditional concept of lunacy covered symptoms wider than the scope of modern psychiatry.

---

8   Quoted in Guthrie D (1948): *A History of Medicine*. London: Thomas Nelson & Sons, p54. Hygeia and Panacea were daughters of Asklepius.

Convulsions are a feature of epilepsy, a condition well known to ancient physicians. The term 'epileptic' is derived from the Greek verb *epilambein*, meaning to seize; as the attacks involved the mind as well as the body, and occurred in regular cycles apparently relating to lunar cycles, the victim was believed to be seized by the Moon. Aristotle thought that children were more prone to epileptic attacks at full moon. For the strength of its muscular contractions, epilepsy was associated with Hercules, but another prominent feature was the expression of pronounced religious ideation around the time of seizures, which led the Greeks and Hebrews to define epilepsy as 'the sacred disease'. As concluded by Hugh Farmer in his *Essay on the Demoniacs of the New Testament* of 1775, it is apparent that persons described as lunatics in the Bible were suffering from epileptic seizures. Matthew, Mark and Luke each told of how Jesus cured an epileptic boy by dispelling an evil spirit. It appears that Jesus distinguished between maladies that were natural diseases, and those caused by diabolical possession, as described in the book of Matthew, Chapter 17:

> And when they were come to the multitude, there came to him a certain man, kneeling down to him, and saying, Lord, have mercy on my son; for he is lunatic, and sore vexed: for ofttimes he falleth into the fire, and oft into the water. And I brought him to thy disciples, and they could not cure him. Then Jesus answered and said, O faithless and perverse generation, how long shall I be with you? How long shall I suffer you? Bring him hither to me. And Jesus rebuked the devil; and he departed out of him: and the child was cured from that very hour.[9]

In Greece, the presentations of epilepsy were attributed to various gods. For example, it was said that nocturnal wanderings were due to the power of Hecate. Sufferers were instructed to avoid wearing black, and treatment included the swallowing of stones, and concoctions of the brains of vultures, the hearts of rabbits, blood from the mortally wounded and human faeces. However, the Hippocratic treatise *On the Sacred Disease* of circa 400BC rejected divine causation, defining epilepsy as a purely physiological disease, with seizures caused by phlegmatic obstruction in the blood vessels of the brain. The writer, probably Hippocrates himself, derided the supernatural interventions of the time, remarked:

> It is my opinion that those who first called this disease 'sacred' were the sort of people we now call witch-doctors, faith-healers, quacks and charlatans. These are exactly the people who pretend to be very pious and to be particularly wise.[10]

The Moon was not mentioned by Hippocrates in relation to epilepsy, but a text from the corpus on dreams illustrates the importance of cosmic influence within the Hippocratic model of natural causation. Moisture

---

9   Gospel according to Matthew, 17:15. King James' Version (2008). London: Collins.
10   Hippocrates (1950): *The Medical Works of Hippocrates* (translated J. Chadwick, Mann WN). Oxford: Blackwell, p179.

was regarded as a key environmental factor in madness, and it was observed that the brains of people with chronic epilepsy were abnormally moist (now known as an accumulation of cerebrospinal fluid). Harmful excretions of fluid into the outer parts of the body were thought to occur when mist or cloud obscured visibility of the Moon and stars. The author stated: 'if the Moon is involved, it is advisable to draw off the matter internally, therefore to use an emetic'.[11] Knowledge of the celestial bodies was thus vital for the physician, as explained in this paragraph:

> It is a healthy sign if any of the heavenly bodies appears clear and moist; because the influx from the aether acting on the person is clear and the mind perceives this as it enters. If it be dark and obscure, then sickness is indicated, not due to some internal excess or lack of something, but coming from the external environment ... It is a good sign to see the Sun, Moon, sky and stars clear and undimmed, each being placed normally in its right place, since it shows that the body is well and free from disturbing influences ... When the heavenly bodies wander in different directions, some mental disturbance as a result of anxiety is indicated.[12]

Greek medicine was certainly not a secular movement. For Plato, the forces of nature were transmitted from the heavens through intelligent celestial essences known as *daemones,* and Aristotle made concessions to occultism by permitting the possibility of cosmic influence on terrestrial life. Prayers to Zeus, Athena, Hermes and Apollo were advised when the cosmic signs were good; and to the Heroes when the stars bade ill. The potential of the Moon to unhinge minds was not doubted, nor was the influence of lunar deity, as in this Hippocratic guidance: 'One who is seized with terror, fright, and madness during the night is being visited by the goddess of the moon.'[13]

The presumed influence of spirits concorded with the humoural model, and this system was further developed by physicians at Alexandria, the seat of Greek medicine from the third century BC onwards. Herophilus (c330–260 BC), who provided convicts for vivisection, observed that the veins and arteries contained blood of differing hue, and that the pulse was governed by the heart. Erististratus (c315–240 BC) defined the heart as a pump that distributed blood to tissues through the veins, but he thought that the arteries carried air (discovery of the circulatory system was for another age). Blood-letting, which had been practised as a sacrificial activity in priestly medicine, was rationalised as an alleviation of humoural excess.

11   Hippocrates (1950), p195.
12   Hippocrates (1950), pp195-198.
13   Quoted by Eysenck HJ and Nias DKB (1982): *Astrology: Science or Superstition?* London: Maurice Temple Smith, p172.

After the collapse of the Hellenistic empire, many Greek physicians worked in Rome. Most prominent was Asclepiades (124 BC–?) of Prusias ad Mare in Bithynia, who practised Methodism, whereby health was determined by a balance between tension and relaxation, regulated by pores throughout body tissue. Among several competing schools in Graeco-Roman medicine were the Dogmatists (vanguards of the Hippocratic tradition), the Empirics (who eschewed theories of causation to focus on treating symptoms), and the Pneumatists (for whom disease of body or soul was caused by bad air). The greatest Roman physician was Claudius Galen (AD 129–199) of Pergamom, who developed Hippocratic medicine into a system that would dominate European medicine for a thousand years.

Court physician to Marcus Aurelius, Galen was primarily an anatomist. He conducted his investigations on the Barbary ape, from which he extrapolated the structures of muscles, brain, blood vessels. He differentiated the sensory and motor branches of the nervous system, and determined the function of the arteries as blood vessels. Galen reinforced the system of four humours. From an expanding pharmacopeia of plant and animal extracts, the practitioner's task was to restore humoural equilibrium, and combinations of substances were selected for their drying, moistening, warming or cooling properties. Displaying his Platonist bent, Galen honoured the tripartite formulation of the spirit, rational thought and basic desires, locating these in the heart, brain, and liver respectively. Together, these parts maintained harmony. His interpretation of the body as merely the vehicle of the soul was later embraced by Christianity, which saw no moral purpose in anatomical study: the body was sacred, and the healer was God.[14] Galen posited the brain as the organ of the mind, and he supported Hippocrates in attributing epilepsy to somatic cause. However, he agreed with scholars such as Aristotle that fits were regulated by the Moon. Galen believed that septenary periodicity in disease, as described in Hippocratic texts, was not due to Pythagorean number lore but to lunar quarters, but he offered no explanation for this effect (although the Moon was related to water, the Greeks failed to establish the tidal connection, possibly because the tidal range is insignificant in the eastern Mediterranean).

A comprehensive assembly of knowledge on the Moon was provided in the first century AD by the prolific pen of Plutarch, a Platonist born in Greece who moved to Rome where he wrote influential philosophical texts. His classic dialogue *De Facie quae in Orbe Lunae Apparet* (*Concerning the Face which Appears on the Orb of the Moon*) combined rational explanation with

---

14 In their opposition to secular teaching, Christians sacked the great library of Alexandria in AD 391. The Greek archives had already been largely destroyed by fire during a first century revolt against Caesar.

fantasy.[15] The Moon was described as an Earth-like domain, and a habitat of humanoid creatures capable of contemplating life on their neighbouring sphere. Among various ideas of lunar influence introduced by Plutarch in the conversation was the belief that by promoting dampness, the Moon boosted growth of plants and animals. Roman encyclopaedist Pliny the Elder (AD 23–79) claimed that the Moon filled and emptied terrestrial bodies as it drew nearer and farther from Earth, and that the volume of blood rose and fell in relation to moonlight. He also wrote that exposure to moonbeams made one liable to become stuporous, with children particularly vulnerable. Ptolemy stated that people with moisture on the brain were susceptible to mental derangement at full moon.

Of all celestial bodies, the Moon was considered to bear strongest influence on health and illness. Traditional teaching had emphasised the divinity of the cosmos, but a distinct lunar influence was incompatible with the rise of monotheism. The Romans tended to accommodate gods of cultures brought into their empire, accepting local deities in their pantheon, but by the second century AD there was a momentum towards worship of a single overarching god. Plotinus (AD 204–270) marked the dawn of neo-Platonism with his concept of 'The One', combining the Aristotlean 'prime mover' with Plato's ultimate good. In AD 274, while Christians were being persecuted, Emperor Aurelian instilled the Assyrian sun god *Deus Sol Invictus* as the supreme Roman deity, but in the following century, encouraged by Constantine, Christianity was established as the official Roman religion. There seemed little in common between the enquiring minds of Athens and the unquestioning faith of Jerusalem. However, Christians embraced the ideal form (if not the ethics) of Plato, the cosmology (but not astrology) of Ptolemy, and the spirit-laden anatomy of the pagan physician Galen. To the Greeks had come the revelation of a mathematical universe, but only Christians appreciated that the spheres were turned by angels. Knowledge was subjugated by institutional religion, whereby all moral and physical laws were imposed by God alone. No longer would people need to fear or worship the Moon.

---

15   Coones P (1983): 'The geographical significance of Plutarch's dialogue, *Concerning the Face which Appears on the Orb of the Moon'. Transactions of the Institute of British Geographers*, 8: 361–372.

Two

The medieval cosmos

Throughout the Middle Ages, madness was a nebulous aspect of the human condition on which physicians, theologians and philosophers mused. The medical interpretation was not of an illness of itself, but as an expression of bodily imbalance. Galenic medicine complemented medieval cosmology, with each humour and its related temperament dominated by a celestial body: the blood and sanguine character by Jupiter and Venus, black bile and melancholia by Saturn, yellow bile and choleric personality by Mars, and phlegm by the Moon. Phlegmatic people were governed by the spiritual element water, their reflective and sensitive nature predisposed to fluctuations in moisture caused by lunar cycles. Whereas Jupiter, the Sun and Venus were inherently benevolent, Saturn, Mars and the Moon were liable to upset the balance of humours and to provoke passions. The Moon was the celestial body most consulted by physicians, for it set the critical periods of mutable diseases; survival to new moon, which was associated with rejuvenation, brought relief. The flow and volume of bodily fluids depended on the position and aspect of the Moon in the zodiac, and barber-surgeons timed their performance of venesection by lunar phase.

Astrology was at the core of the prospectus at the fledgling universities of western Europe, where budding physicians learned how planetary properties and motions predicted character, vigour and disease. A standard feature of medical books was the illustrated 'zodiac man', with Aries, first sign of the astrological year, governing the head; the feet were in the dominion of Pisces. Instead of the natal horoscope, physicians often drew the chart on the hour of 'decumbiture' (when the patient was struck with illness). However, the status of astrology in Christendom was contentious. Saint Augustine of Hippo (354–430) had taught that magic, starlore and fortune-telling contradicted the omnipotence of God and the doctrine of free will; while the stars governed aspects of nature, for humankind, faith was all that mattered. Fearing the return of Paganism, the Church officially regarded astrology as false idolatry, and it was intended that saints of specific diseases would replace the zodiacal model; epilepsy, for example, was under patronage of Saint Christopher. In 1108 the Archbishop of York was refused Christian burial after a book on astrology was found under his pillow. By contrast, Pope Leo X founded a professorship in the subject at the University of Rome, as did several other centres of scholasticism. Most theologians accepted a limited astral influence, analogous to the effect of wind on a ship's course: the stars incline, but do not compel. Fate and Providence were thus uncomfortable bedfellows, a compromise of traditional beliefs and revealed truth.

Measurement and meaning

While Christendom languished in Platonist dogma, the Arabs, who had inherited the Alexandrian archives, had made great strides in scientific enquiry. They laid the foundations of chemistry and algebra, and refined the axiomatic geometry of Euclid. Astronomy had practical benefit to the Islamic world, as knowledge of celestial patterns aided orientation in a barren landscape, followers being required to bow towards Mecca five times per day. Moslem scholars improved the astrolabe, an ancient forerunner of the pocket watch, which determined the time of day from the relative positions of the Sun and stars. Some gaps were filled in Ptolemy's work, including the Andromeda galaxy, which to the keen naked eye appears as a cloud. A legacy of Arab astronomy is in terms such as 'azimuth', 'zenith' and 'nadir'. Geocentrism was cemented in Islam, but believers were encouraged to marvel at the heavens.

The Moon attracted much interest from Arab astronomers. Mohammed ben Jabir al-Battani, or Albategnius (858–929) refined Ptolemy's calculations of the lunar orbit (one of the largest craters is named after him). Al-Hasanibn al-Haytham (965–1039), also known as Alhazen, produced two observational texts on the nearest sphere: *On the Light of the Moon*, and *On the Nature of the Marks Seen on the Surface of the Moon*. Just as the Christians have the cross and the Jews the Star of David, the crescent moon is associated with Islam. When the Turks conquered Constantinople in 1453, the crescent moon symbol of the ancient city (which reputedly honoured lunar goddess Diana) was adopted by the Ottoman Empire, and became an unofficial motif of the Mohammedan religion.

In the twelfth century, the classic works of Greek natural philosophy filtered from Moorish to Christian Spain. The treasures of knowledge were brought from Arabic into Latin, including Ptolemy's *Almagest*, translated at the great library of Toledo in 1175. Some texts featured commentary from their Arab guardians. Renowned for his cogent discussion of Aristotle was philosopher and physician Averroës (1126–1198). Born in Córdova in Moorish Spain, Averroës is somewhat unfairly associated with the 'double truth' of theological and material knowledge, to which western historians have attributed the decline in Islamic science. Averroës was a determinist who espoused the Aristotlean idea of an eternal universe, and adherents to his philosophy were censored by the Church. A satisfactory resolution of the conflict between faith and reason was presented in the profound cosmological argument of aristocratic Dominican monk Thomas Aquinas (1225–1274), whose *Summa Theologica* applied Aristotle's concept of a prime mover as the rationale for Christian belief. Aquinas argued that as God's existence must have preceded his essence, he must present pure existence. Knowledge could only be derived through God's creation; in harmony, faith and reason led to one truth. This stance, endorsed by the Catholic Church, licensed tentative progress in natural philosophy. God wrote the laws of nature, and observation or reasoning could only illuminate his perfect design.

Not only did the medieval Church hold humanity together through the turbulence of wars, pestilence and famine, but major contributions to knowledge emerged from its institutes of learning, as James Hannam eloquently illuminated in his book *God's Philosophers*. In the neat narrative of popular history, the schoolmen of the so-called Dark Ages stood diametrically opposed to scientific enquiry, controlling knowledge to bolster the hegemony of the Church. Much emphasis has been placed on a few controversial scholars who were tortured or executed for heresy, but in fact scholars had much latitude for conjecture and debate; indeed, the principle of academic freedom originated in the medieval university. Technical advances included the mechanical clock and spectacles, and development of the magnetic compass. In the fourteenth century a succession of scholars at Oxford University known as the 'Merton Calculators' dislodged the pillars of Aristotle's laws of motion. An emerging empiricism was characterised by Roger Bacon (1214–1294). Whereas the works of Greek scholars contained few mathematical formulae, Bradwardine (c1290–1349) emphasised measurement in natural philosophy, pointing the way to modern scientific method: 'Whoever has the effrontery to pursue physics while neglecting mathematics should know from the start that he will never make his entry through the portals of wisdom.'[1]

Despite the pedestal on which Aristotlean physics sat, it became increasingly evident that classical knowledge was not the final say on physical phenomena, particularly in the domain of astronomy. The completeness and accuracy of Ptolemy's text had required improvement by Moslem

---

1   Quoted in Molland AG (1968): 'The geometrical background to the Merton School'. *British Journal for the History of Science*, 4. p110.

scholars. In the late thirteenth century, Alfonso X (The Wise) employed fifty foreign astronomers at Castile, mostly Arabs, on the refinement of planetary tables. Taken aback by the complexity of the Ptolemaic system, the sovereign reputedly exclaimed: 'Had God consulted me during the Creation, I would have recommended a simple structure to him.'[2]

Astronomy was the first mathematical science, forming part of the *quadrivium* alongside arithmetic, geometry and music (these subjects were of lower status than the *trivium* of logic, grammar and rhetoric). The objective was to describe rather than explain celestial motions. While it was widely believed that human and terrestrial phenomena were subject to celestial influence, this was the domain of the horoscope, not of numerical measurement.

Among the general populace, the stars were seen as messengers of divine wrath. At predicted conjunctions of planetary courses, underground shelters were dug in preparation for the anticipated Biblical tempests, as occurred in the years 1229, 1236, 1339, 1371, 1395, 1422, 1432, 1451, 1460 and 1487. Comets were regarded as prophecies of doom. Venerable Bede (673–735) had warned that such projectiles 'portend revolution of kingdoms, pestilence, war, winds or heat'[3], and the Bayeux Tapestry depicts King Harold being foretold of his fate as a comet flies overhead. Tragic events occurred frequently enough to be linked to a recent celestial event, and scholars did little to assuage public scare.

In the late Middle Ages much academic energy was expended on the occult, which basically meant any hidden phenomena, such as magic or magnetism, and astrology gained credibility following the translation of Ptolemy's *Tetrabiblios*. Regiomontanus (1436–1476, born Johannes Müller), distinguished professor of astronomy at the University of Vienna, was a prominent astrologer who devised the *Modus Rationalis* method of house division.[4] The uncannily accurate prophet Michael Nostradamus (1503–1566), born at St Remy in Provence, emphasised astrological knowledge in medicine. Historians of psychiatry Hunter and Macalpine remarked:

> That astrology survived so long seems less absurd when it is remembered that at that time man knew more about the macrocosm and the laws governing the heavenly bodies than about the microcosm and the workings of his own.[5]

2   Quoted by Rudolf Thiel (1958): *And There Was Light*, p73.
3   Quoted by Bertrand Russell (1952/1994): *The Impact of Science on Society*. London: Routledge, pp13-14.
4   Like many humanist scholars, Müller classicised his name.
5   Hunter R, Macalpine I (1963): *Three Hundred Years of Psychiatry 1535–1860*. London: Oxford University Press, p141.

Paracelsian medicine

Cosmic influence on health was a dominant theme of the maverick physician Philippus Aureolus Theophrastus Bombast von Hohenheim (1493–1541), who named himself Paracelsus. Following his successful treatment of humanist publisher Frobenius of Basle, whose leg he saved from amputation, Paracelsus was appointed town physician and university lecturer in medicine at Basle. Pouring scorn on Galenic medicine, he symbolically hurled the standard medical textbook of Avicenna (980–1036), the great Persian physician, into the bonfire at the annual student gala. Paracelsus impressed on trainees his 'Four Pillars of Medicine': philosophy, virtue (meaning the healing power of astral essence), alchemy and astronomy (as conflated with astrology). His astro-alchemical model was never widely accepted, but his historical importance arises from his radical assertion that physical or mental disturbance was not caused by aberrant humours but by distinct diseases — for which specific remedies could be found.

Like Hippocrates, Paracelsus denied supernatural causation, but he was a mystic nonetheless. Eschewing the traditional pharmacopeia of plant derivatives, his treatments were a practical application of alchemy, the body of knowledge relating metals and other substances to human life. Originating in ancient Egypt, alchemy was given a semblance of rationale by early Greek philosophers in their cogitations on a primordial substance. Alchemy was tied to the system of four elements, and to these material substances Arab scholars added two philosophical elements. Mercury, the dense, permanent substance, contrasted with the inflammable, transient sulphur; with this combination, metals were formed. Medieval scholars such as Roger Bacon believed that such *materia prima* was obtainable through removal of impurities. Indeed, the ultimate prize of alchemy was to obtain from base metal the precious, incorruptible gold. To mercury and sulphur Paracelsus added salt, believing that all three spiritual elements were essential to transmutation.

The Moon was a potent cosmic agent for alchemists, who believed that purer metals could be obtained by working under a waxing luminary, due to increased moisture. Paracelsian medicine required correct timing for preparation of chemical remedies, to obtain the quintessence of favourably positioned stars. Reviving ancient numerary logic, Paracelsus linked the seven planets with the seven principal metals: gold with the Sun, mercury with its namesake, iron with Mars, tin with Jupiter, lead with Saturn and copper with Venus; the cold Moon hosted silver.[6] The 'mysterium', the intermediary between Earth and the heavens, was the conduit of an aethereal spirit, which pervaded the cosmos and exerted influence throughout the sublunary domain. The relationship of human microcosm to ambient macrocosm was through the elements mercury, sulphur and salt. Mercury represented the emotions, based in the heart; sulphur drove the will and sexuality; salt was the thinking component, regulated by lunar forces. Each organ related to a planet: the heart to the Sun, the spleen to Saturn, the liver to Jupiter, and the brain to the Moon. As the source of all energy, celestial bodies could provoke or relieve illness, although such power was not deterministic — Paracelsus avoided heretical denial of free will. Talismanic magic was applied in the wearing of amulets containing the apprpriate essence. In some conditions Paracelsian medicine had proven results. Celestial association with metals led to the notable discovery that mercury could cure syphilis. The Martian element, iron, Paracelsus claimed, benefited patients suffering deficiency in the blood. He claimed that if a man was agitated, the likely cause was not excessive bile, as conventional physicians would explain, but provocation by Mars.

Attracting ridicule from medical peers for his wild ideas and self-aggrandisement, Paracelsus was repeatedly refused publication. However, his influence grew in the decades after his death, and he became known as the 'Luther of medicine'. Although his posthumously published works were laden with piety and mysticism, Paracelsus emphasised the healing powers of nature, albeit within a speculative cosmic system. Among his dozens of medical books was *Diseases that Deprive Man of his Reason*, which described lunatics as suffering from a fluctuating form of madness, whose *spiritus vitae cerebri*, just like the needle of the compass, was attracted to the North Pole. According to Paracelsus their ravings occurred most frequently at new moon, when the strength of magnetic pull aroused sexual passions, and brought disturbing dreams and hallucinations. Some people, he observed, were more vulnerable to lunar influence: 'The *spiritus sensitivus* of a man who is weak and offers no resistance may be attracted toward the moon and be poisoned by its evil influence.'[7] As well as calming unruly passions by applying magnetic iron, Paracelsus treated lunatics with extracts of plants of lunar association such as *Helleborus niger* and *Thymus majorana*, and amulets of silver. However, he also espoused the more instant remedy of plunging the madman in cold water.

6   Analysis of a soil sample from an American rocket probe piercing the Cabeus crater has revealed that silver actually exists on the Moon, as reported in Schultz PH, Hermalyn B, Colaprete A, Ennico K, Shirley M, Marshall WS (2010): 'The LCROSS Cratering Experiment'. *Science*, 330: 468–472.
7   Quoted in Oliven (1943).

The Copernican revolution

According to popular history, the spirit of enquiry dramatically returned in the Renaissance of the fifteenth and sixteenth centuries. However, this retrospectively-defined movement was not discrete in duration or impact, and one must be wary of the Whiggish historicism noted by Henry Butterfield, whereby a complex interplay of philosophical, theological and socio-political forces is conveniently reduced to a narrative of linear progress.[8] The Renaissance was not a primer for atheism but a conservative movement. Striving for erudition in the authentic wisdom of classical civilisation, humanist scholars discarded medieval literature as corruption of ancient texts. The style of Plato trumped the substance of Aristotle, and the mysticism of Pythagoras was preferred to the logic and observations of more recent scholarship.

The humanist assertions of Machiavelli and Erasmus, emergence of an educated mercantile class in the burgeoning city states, and wider circulation of books enabled by the printing press — many factors combined to loosen the ecclesiastical hold on knowledge. Festering dissent against Church dogma eventually burst out in the Reformation of the sixteenth century. In 1517 German priest Martin Luther nailed ninety-five statements to the church door at Wittenberg, opposing papal ornament and 'indulgences', whereby people paid money forgiveness of sin. In his treatise *The Freedom of a Christian Man*, Luther promoted the Pauline doctrine of personal communication with God, whose truth was to be found through introspection. Luther was excommunicated, but gained such support that a new church was founded in his name. A more extreme attack on the Catholic Church was led by Ulrich Zwingli, whose Programme of Reform of 1523 led to civil war in Switzerland. In the 1540s John Calvin, having gained support in France, Germany and Holland, established another Protestant church in Geneva. Although the Reformation liberated people from Rome, it did not produce a single unified authority. Dismantling of the old regime in northern Europe was followed by fierce competition between denominations, each claiming to represent true faith. The Counter Reformation and ensuing strife escalated to decades of warfare across Europe, eventually dividing Europe into Protestant north and Catholic south.

In the spirit of neo-Platonist humanism, before the strictures of Inquisition and religious fanaticism, a novel cosmological idea was presented by

8   Butterfield H (1931): *The Whig Interpretation of History*. London: Bell.

Cardinal Nicholas of Cusa (1400–1464). His widely read thesis *On Learned Ignorance* argued that humankind should accept the limits to knowledge. The author felt confident in the majesty of God to postulate an infinite universe, in which Earth itself was constantly in motion. Meanwhile Georg Peurbach, an acquaintance of the cardinal, began a translation of Ptolemy's original Greek text, of which a copy had been rescued by Christian scholars fleeing Constantinople. This work was continued by his assistant Regiomontanus, whose recalculation of Ptolemy's tables revealed various anomalies, including an eclipse that occurred eleven minutes earlier than predicted by the Alexandrian master. Ptolemy's system was good, but not quite good enough. The stage was set for an inquisitive Polish priest to begin an intellectual revolution that would bring an end to medieval cosmology.

Nicolaus Copernicus (1473–1543, born Mikolaj Kopernik) went to the university at Cracow and from there to Bologna, initially to study ecclesiastical law. In the relatively cloudless Mediterranean climate, Copernicus was able to pursue his passion in astronomy, and with a generous stipend from his rich uncle, he spent ten years at the prestigious universities of northern Italy. Appreciating the problems of the Ptolemaic system, Copernicus put his enquiring mind to the challenge of devising a more viable model. He trawled ancient texts and found two fundamental ideas, dismissed by Ptolemy, but worthy of reconsideration. Firstly, there was the notion that the Earth spun on its axis. Cicero had recorded the belief of Nicetas of Syracuse that the Earth rotated, while all other celestial bodies were stationary. This could not be right, as the Moon and Sun obviously moved in relation to each other. Ptolemy had argued that if Earth span in one direction, the winds must always blow the other way. However, Copernicus surmised that as Earth rotated, so would its enveloping atmosphere.

The second idea not satisfactorily refuted by Ptolemy, was that Earth moved in space. Copernicus may not have seen the heliocentric argument of Aristarchus, a translated text not appearing in western Europe until after his death, but he would have been aware from other Greek authors of the idea of the Sun as the central source of warmth and light, circulated by Earth and the planets. Intrigued by the possibility of solar dominion, Copernicus developed a model of planetary orbits of varying lengths. Mars, for example, with an orbit twice as wide as that of Earth, would take two years to circulate the Sun. With a system that complied with most observations, the multitude of epicycles and eccentrics were obviated. However, the thesis was also likely to be considered heretical. Copernicus had his treatise *De Revolutionibus Orbium Caelestium* prefaced by Andreas Osiander, a Lutheran minister, who described the thesis not as a statement of reality, but as a mathematical device for calculating planetary movements. To avoid retribution, Copernicus withheld publication until he was safely deceased.

The Copernican model was largely ignored by the religious censors, and indeed by fellow astronomers. Only a thousand copies were initially printed, and its small readership was probably due to how awkwardly Copernicus presented his thesis; a straightforward idea was mired in a cumbersome reworking of the Ptolemaic wheeled universe. A forgiving reader was Thomas Digges (1546–1595). He supported the heliocentric theory in *A Perfit Description of the Caelestiall Orbes*, published as an appendix to his father's almanac in 1576, which speculated an infinite universe of countless stars. William Gilbert (1544–1603), in his classic text *De Magnete*, proposed magnetism as the force maintaining the planets in orbit of the Sun. However, the most prominent astronomer of the late sixteenth century, Tycho Brahe (1546–1601), upheld the geocentric universe.

Court astrologer to the Danish monarchy, Tycho received ample support from King Frederick II, and was handed the island of Hven in the Baltic Sea, where he built a palatial edifice lavishly equipped with instruments for celestial measurement.[9] Rejecting speculative cosmological theories, Tycho asserted that no proposition was credible without systematic observation. The most meticulous observer of the cosmos since Hipparchus, Tycho's interest in astronomy was kindled by two events. In 1563 the timing of an anticipated near-conjunction of Jupiter and Saturn showed that neither the system of Ptolemy nor Copernicus predicted planetary motions satisfactorily. In 1572 a bright star had appeared in the W-shaped constellation Cassiopeia, drawing great public interest (some astrologers suggested the return of the Star of Bethlehem). For eighteen months it was visible in daylight. Now known to have been a supernova, this celestial body, absent from the Greek records, shattered the notion of an eternal firmament. Furthermore, in 1577 Tycho observed a comet moving across the distant spheres of the planets, far beyond the supposed atmospheric domain of such projectiles. Tycho was a pompous character, and on making an enemy of himself in Denmark, he took up residence in Prague, under the Habsburg empire, where he continued his work. He developed a widely accepted system whereby Sun and Moon revolved around a static Earth, with the planets moving around the Sun. On theoretical and theological grounds, Tycho could not accept that the Earth was in orbit or spin.

Neither the heliocentric hypothesis nor the model of Tycho permitted the fixed spheres of classical cosmology. Believing that he could improve the Copernican system, mathematician Johannes Kepler (1571–1630) looked beyond geometry for a causal explanation for the planetary

---

9   When Shakespeare was writing *The Tempest*, he would have known of the visit by King James to the Hven observatory, and Tycho was almost certainly the inspiration for the character Prospero.

motions, thereby introducing physics to astronomy. Noting that Mercury was the fastest planet and closest to the Sun, and that Saturn was slowest and farthest away, Kepler attributed the planetary orbits to solar attraction. This progression from 'how' to 'why' was not punished in the relatively tolerant atmosphere of Graz in Austria, where Kepler taught mathematics and astronomy, but after his Lutheran school was closed down by order of Archduke Ferdinand, in 1600 he accepted an invitation to become Tycho's assistant in Prague. On his deathbed, Tycho at last gave Kepler access to his treasured records, which could now be fully exploited.

The heliocentric hypothesis was most frustrated by Mars, which seemed to decelerate during its cycle, and this planet was the subject of many months of calculations by Kepler. Eventually, Kepler deduced that instead of a circular motion, each planet revolved in an ellipse, with speed varying at different stages of the journey, but covering the same area of arc. This discovery did not fit his initial hypothesis that the planetary orbits were caused by magnetism, so he speculated that the elongated cycles must be the result of antagonistic forces. His *Astronomia Nova* was published in 1609, with the full, poignant title translated as *A New Astronomy Based on Causation, or a Physics of the Sky, derived from Investigations of the Motions of the star Mars, founded on Observations of the noble Tycho Brahe*. Kepler's model offered an escape from circular dogma, but received a cool reception. However, long before releasing his *magnum opus*, Kepler had drawn interest from Galileo Galilei (1564–1642), then a professor of mathematics at Padua.

An intellectual rebel, Galileo set out to disprove all elements of Aristotlean physics, and he finally refuted the enduring idea that the speed of a falling object was determined by its weight. Galileo eschewed the contemplative knowledge of traditional scholarship to assert that theory should match experience, and this required rigorous testing of hypotheses. Famously, he described mathematics as the language of the Universe. Galileo was also aware of the dangers of asserting ideas at odds with Christian doctrine, as demonstrated in the Roman Inquisition case against Giordano Bruno (1548–1600). An outspoken critic of Catholic doctrine, Bruno followed the cult of Hermes Trismegistus, whose ancient Egyptian mysticism had honoured the Sun as the centre of the cosmos. The Copernican system, while denounced by Luther as contradiction of Scripture, had not troubled the Catholic Church, being merely a proposition that could be casually dismissed. Bruno went further, describing an infinite universe with many solar systems and habitable planets; he also denied the virgin birth and described Jesus as mere magician. A perpetual thorn in the side of the authorities, Bruno was burnt at the stake. Although heliocentrism was not the only reason for this execution, Galileo was understandably cautious in expressing support for the Copernican model.

However, the greatest obstacle was his academic superiors at Padua, who were staunch disciples of Aristotle and Ptolemy.

So far, astronomy had relied on the naked eye, but in the late sixteenth century the potential of a double lens to magnify distant objects was coming to light. In 1608 Dutch spectacle-maker Hans Lippershey combined a convex and a concave lens to produce a telescopic device. His was not the first, Leonard Digges (according to his astronomer son Thomas) having derived amusement from a similar tool twenty years earlier. However, Lippershey obtained a patent by the Dutch establishment, and went on to market his telescopes across Europe. An early object of telescopic interest was the Moon. The imaginative Leonardo da Vinci had noted in 1490 the possibility of 'making glasses to see the Moon enlarged',[10] and this feat was first realised in 1609 by English polymath Thomas Harriot. Looking through his basic 'Dutch trunke' telescope from his house at Syon Park in Middlesex, he drew maps of the lunar surface. Once Galileo heard of the invention he quickly produced his own improvised apparatus, with a magnification factor of twenty; it generated great interest on public display in Venice. For all the wisdom of the Greek scholars and their Arab successors, their knowledge was limited by natural sensory capacity; it was the telescope that established the symbiosis of science and technology.

In 1610, in the pamphlet *Siderius Nuncius* (*Messenger from the Stars*), the first publication of telescopic astronomy, Galileo revealed astounding details about the near and distant universe, as seen for the first time. He described the rough lunar terrain, detecting mountains and valleys from the presence of shadows, proving that the Moon was no perfect sphere. Venus was found to change from full disc to a crescent, and by following the position of sunspots, Galileo discovered the rotation of the Sun. Most significantly, he identified four moons in orbit of Jupiter, which finally debunked the idea that all celestial orbits were centred on Earth, and also showed that our own Moon was not unique. Here was validation of the Copernican system, although Galileo was careful to avoid saying so. However, he incriminated himself by overtly challenging religious givens in a widely distributed letter to his former pupil, the Benedictine priest Castelli, now professor of mathematics at Pisa. In 1616 the Copernican thesis was added to the Index of Forbidden Books, and the authorities warned Galileo that he could teach as an idea, but not defend it. Otherwise Galileo was free to continue his scientific endeavours, and his work on dynamics proved useful to the military. His theory of perpetual motion was an important stepping stone in explaining Kepler's ellipses.

---

10 Quoted in Whitehouse D (2003): *The Moon: A Biography*. London: Headline, p56. However, da Vinci's notebooks containing his scientific insights were not discovered until centuries later.

Kepler and Galileo were contemporaries, but after first corresponding in 1597, their communication was sporadic, as the latter often failed to reciprocate. Galileo also displayed lapses in scientific attitude, mocking his German colleague for attributing the ocean tides to lunar cycles. Galileo continued to assert that tides were caused by the rotation of Earth, and jibed that Kepler should spend less time with his horoscopes. Indeed, Kepler regularly issued a calendar of astrological forecasts, supplementing his meagre salary at Graz, and was later court astrologer to the Duke of Wallenstein. His mysticism was unleashed in the work *Harmonices Mundi* of 1619, in which the musical scale was derived from the diurnal heliocentric angles of the planets. Kepler considered the influence of stellar constellations a valid matter for enquiry, and while he was no apologist for popular astrology, he acknowledged the debt of astronomy to its shadow pursuit: 'for a hundred years past, this wise mother could not have lived without the help of her foolish daughter'.[11]

Kepler also wrote what some writers credit as the first science-fiction story, his unfinished *Somnium sive Opus Posthuman de Astronomia Sublunari* (*Dream of the Moon*).[12] In this offering, a bridge formed by the shadow of Earth on each lunar eclipse allowed human passage to the Moon. A return journey was only possible at solar eclipse, by similar means. Kepler described how space travellers were suspended by a balance of the magnetic forces of Earth and Moon, thus hinting at universal gravitation. The strange beasts of the Moon were entirely nocturnal, sheltering in the daytime from the blistering sun in great caves. The craters, in this imaginary tale, were built by the lunar creatures.

The seventeenth century saw a boom in selenography, as astronomers rushed to chart our nearest and most intriguing celestial body. The Moon was generally believed to contain seas and continents. Galileo did not dispute the existence of lunar oceans, but he reported only what he saw. He was not the first cartographer of the Moon, William Gilbert having produced a detailed map in 1600. The outstanding lunar atlas was produced by Johannes Hevelius (1611–1687), son of a wealthy Danzig brewer, who built a well-equipped observatory, and the longest telescope yet produced. Hevelius published his *Selenographia* in 1647, in which he named 275 features. Details of the Moon were often named after national leaders, but such virtual colonisation was unsustainable. A universally accepted nomenclature was presented by Giovanni Battista Riccioli (1598–1671), Jesuit priest and professor of natural philosophy, first at Padua and then at

---

11   Hone ME (1978): *The Modern Text-Book of Astrology* (revised edition). Romford: LN Fowler, p293.

12   The first fictional moon adventure was by Lucian of Samosata (AD 120–180), whose satirical *Vera Historia* told of men caught in a whirlwind landing on the Moon, which was then at war with the Sun. The moon warriors rode on giant fleas and their diet was roast frogs.

Bologna. In 1651 Riccioli's *Almagestum Novum* was published as a rebuttal of Copernicanism, but on his lunar map he honoured the great astronomers, alongside several saints. The legendary influences of the Moon were immortalised by the naming of the seas of tranquillity, fertility, cold and rain, and — in *Mare Crisium* — madness.

Current writers often attribute to the pioneers of modern science a direct opposition to the religious establishment. Yet Kepler was a man of strong faith, whose calculations revealed that God had no reason to steer the stars, because his creation ran like clockwork. However, Galileo was provocative, and eventually stretched the tolerance of the religious authorities too far. The required neutrality on heliocentrism was found lacking by censors in his *Diologo* (*Dialogue Concerning the Two Chief Systems of the World*), which presented a debate between a Copernican, an Aristotlean and a layman. Mischievously, he named the Aristotlean scholar Simplicio, perhaps after an actual sixth-century natural philosopher of that tradition, but it implied simple-mindedness. Worse still, the words spoken by Simplicio repeated those of Pope Urban VIII in earlier communication. The book was completed in 1630 without the recommended preface, and on applying for the requisite papal permission to publish, Galileo was summoned by the Inquisition. At the trial he pleaded guilty to a charge of heresy, thus avoiding torture, and was placed under house arrest at his villa in Florence. The *Dialogue* was smuggled out of the country and published in the Lutheran north, but the Catholic Church maintained its opposition to the heliocentric model for centuries to come.

The rise and fall of spiritual possession

Superstition was not swept aside by the scientific revolution. Outside the university, the populace of Europe had access to a proliferation of vernacular texts on spiritual and occult knowledge. Post-Renaissance alchemy and astrology developed as technical arts, their practitioners claiming the ability to manipulate the hidden powers of magic. Occultism was encouraged by the spirit of neo-Platonism in academe, and astrologers such as Alberti strove to reconcile developments in mathematical theory with the Pythagorean concept of celestial harmony. Scientific advances had explained *how*, but not *why* , and the underlying meaning of phenomena was a matter of ongoing debate in theological circles. The pot of demonology had been simmering for some time, but spilled over in the religious turmoil of the sixteenth and seventeenth centuries. The stance of late medieval theologians oscillated between spiritual communication being illusory, and concern that diabolical interference was a genuine danger to Christendom. Pagan rituals and beliefs in magic and witchcraft were increasingly associated with the Devil. The Church referred to Saint Augustine's conception of demons as eternal spirits who sought to induce human reverence, thus luring people from *civitate dei* to *civitas diaboli*. Cases of apparent demoniacal communication were treated by priests, with occult intervention sometimes summoned to exorcise a malevolent spirit, but a harsher attitude emerged in the late Middle Ages.

In 1484 a papal bull of Innocent VIII endorsed the persecutory zeal of friar Heinrich Kramer, whose *Malleus Maleficarum* (*Witches' Hammer*) of 1486 became the authoritative manual for prosecuting witches. The fleeting tolerance of the Renaissance was replaced by fear and suspicion at every level of society. Witch hunts spread throughout Europe at a time of religious and political strife, epidemic diseases, and the cold weather of a minor ice age and consequent crop failures. To Calvinists and Lutherans, the mischief of the Devil was omnipresent, and radical sects cited the instruction from *Exodus,* Chapter 22, in the Old Testament: 'Thou shalt not suffer a witch to live'. It became heresy to deny the existence of demons. Many thousands of alleged witches and sorcerers were summarily tried and executed. The mother of Kepler narrowly escaped such fate, being shown leniency and imprisoned. Kepler feared that he had contributed to her prosecution, because in his fictional journey to the Moon, she had cast a spell allowing such travel. Martin Luther believed himself to have been visited by demons, and the great humanist Erasmus saw witchcraft as a genuine phenomenon.

The persecuted were mostly impoverished older women, but anyone displaying strange behaviour was endangered. Oliver Temkin's history of epilepsy told how the syndrome commonly known as the 'falling sickness', was termed *morbus demoniacus* ('falling evil') by Luther and others.[13] Around the time of attacks, victims were known to speak in strange tongues. In a tract on epilepsy in 1602, French physician Jean Taxil stated that in nearly all cases of demoniacal possession, seizures occurred. Nonetheless, by diagnosing idiopathic epilepsy, physicians saved many an innocent life. Spiritual possession was compatible with Galenic medicine, which considered disease as a foreign incursion to be expelled by bleeding or purging, just as a demon might be exorcised by a priest. Indeed, illness was implicitly identified with sin, and as divine retribution. Jean Fernel, professor of medicine in Paris, believed that the Devil could turn man into beast, while Ambroise Paré, renowned sixteenth century surgeon, urged execution of anyone claiming magical powers.

---

13   Temkin O (1971): *The Falling Sickness* (2nd edition). Baltimore: John Hopkins Press.

Despite swearing by the Hippocratic Oath, with its dictum *primum non nocere* (first, do no harm), physicians accepted that drastic measures were required in cases of demoniacal possession. However, some learned men raised their heads above the parapet to plead that witches were victims rather than wilful accomplices of evil spirits, urging a more sympathetic response. In 1518, through the perseverance of Agrippa von Nettesheim (1486–1535), legal advisor to the city of Metz, a woman was acquitted on a charge of witchcraft. Agrippa, a leading scholar of occultism, claimed that brutality against allegedly bewitched women was an affront to Christianity, but his stance brought him into conflict with the town inquisitor. While Agrippa was ostracised, his courageous stance inspired his pupil Johann Weyer (1515–1588).

As a physician, Weyer applied his diagnostic expertise to investigate the evidence put forward in witchcraft cases. He observed that the features described in the *Malleus Maleficarum* were really symptoms of mental disorder, having natural rather than supernatural causes. Despite being romanticised as a rational pioneer of psychiatry, Weyer did not deny the presence of the Devil; for example, he described instances of individuals regurgitating a bolus of foreign material such as wool or nails, which apparently could only have been ingested by dark means. However, his denouncement of witch trials, *De Praestiglis Daemonium* (*The Deception of Demons*), published in 1563, was a rebuttal of institutional terror. Nonetheless, local jurists ignored him and continued their prosecutions. Another damning critique appeared in 1584, Reginald Scot's *Discoverie of Witchcraft* the product of the author's horror at summary trials in Kent. This book incurred the wrath of King James VI of Scotland (1566–1625), who was personally involved in cases during his reign in a country of widespread belief in witchcraft. In 1597 his treatise *Daemonology* reinforced the need for radical intervention, even commending the ancient and generally abandoned custom of ducking the accused as a test of guilt (if they drowned, they were innocent). In 1604, shortly after being crowned James I of England, he passed a law stiffening the punishment for witches.

Pivotal in medieval magic, the Moon was closely linked to witchcraft. The *Malleus Maleficarum* stated that demons relied on the forces of nature as a medium for their evil powers, and that they 'molest men at certain phases of the Moon'. Lunar quarters determined when to work spells and to summon fairies.[14] It was believed that witches congregated at full moon, when they sometimes conspired with werewolves. The expansive forestry of medieval Europe supported a large population of wolves, which continued to be feared as predators, with their eerily silent movement, sinister slanting eyes and a terrifying howl that was considered an omen of death.

---

14   Johnson M (2006): 'The Moon'. In *Encyclopedia of Witchcraft: the Western Tradition* (ed. RM Golden). Santa Barbara, California: ABC-CLIO, 781–783.

Pliny the Elder had noted in his *Natural History* that one member of each generation of a family was destined to spend nine years as a nocturnal wolf. Some people strove to become a werewolf, often to exact revenge. Witches performed the transformation ritual at full moon, when a magic circle was formed around a fire heating a cauldron containing a potion of herbs and drugs. The prospective werewolf smeared his or her body with an ointment made from a freshly killed cat, mixed with other ingredients such as opium and aniseed, tied a wolfskin belt around the waist, then kneeled to recite an incantation to the Wolf Spirit.[15] In France, thirty thousand cases of lycanthropy were identified between 1520 and 1630. A notorious case was tried in Cologne in 1589. Under torture, Peter Stumpf confessed that at the age of twelve the devil had given him a magic belt, enabling his metamorphosis into a ferocious wolf. His feeding frenzy over a period of twenty-five years included thirteen children and two pregnant women, whose foetuses he tore from the womb to devour, as well as various livestock. In a punishment of exemplary cruelty, Stumpf was tied to a wheel, his flesh removed by red-hot pincers, his limbs broken, before he was beheaded and burned. Deemed accomplices, his daughter and a mistress were also reduced to ashes.

Testimony of a physician was often sought in cases of alleged witchcraft; William Harvey, for example, was asked to examine several women accused of raising a storm at sea off the west coast of Scotland that had imperilled the king. The absence of physical signs of diabolical incursion saved many women from condemnation. Yet physicians, like judges, practised in a culture where the Devil was fundamental as an opposite to Christian faith. The potential for demoniacal possession was thus generally accepted. However, by the late seventeenth century, the credibility of evil spirits was waning, as it was not supported by medical examination. An increasingly formalised judiciary was less willing to convict on the presented evidence, and by emphasising the omnipotence of God, theologians helped to reduce the panic. Louis XIV abolished the death penalty for witchcraft in France in 1682. Witchcraft, and the extremism of radical preachers, were reinterpreted as madness.

As Nicholas Campion explains, astrology was not compatible with witchcraft, demoniacal and celestial influence being quite different explanations for deviance, yet astrologers were often consulted to investigate suspected bewitchment.[16] Learned English statesman Francis Bacon (1561–1626), although best known for his manifesto of empiricism, wrote *Astrologica Sana*, explaining how the zodiac governed the fate of royalty and commoner alike. As Allan Chapman explained in his account of astro-

15   Farson D, Hall A (1991): *Mysterious Monsters*. London: Bloomsbury.
16   Campion N (2006): 'Astrology'. In *Encyclopedia of Witchcraft: the Western Tradition* (ed. RM Golden). Santa Barbara, California: ABC-CLIO, 64–65.

logical medicine, although its results were dubious, this was no more so than for standard Galenic practice.[17] In his *Astrologicall Judgement of Diseases* of 1655, medically-trained herbalist Nicholas Culpeper (1616–1654) asserted that mental and bodily ills were affected by the Sun, Moon and other planets. Culpeper argued that 'only astrologers are fit to study medicine and a medical man without astrology is like a lamp without oil'.[18] Influenza was so named by the Italians on being attributed to astral malevolence. Many popular almanacs were written by physicians, featuring zodiac man, times for bleeding and purging and a basic medical astrology. With its bewildering complexity, and with growing scepticism about its prognostic value, the role of astrology in medicine declined. By the early seventeenth century it had disappeared from serious medical texts.

With some impressive curative results, alchemy outlived the zodiac in medical occultism. Well into the seventeenth century, an undercurrent of Paracelsian medicine flowed against the Galenic mainstream. Alchemical practice, however, was only partially empirical, remaining steeped in Hermetic mysticism, as historian Charles Webster explained: 'The medical relevance of alchemy lies not simply in its practical concern with chemical therapy, but also in the aim to create a total and harmonious relationship between man and the universe.'[19] Even without reference to astrology and alchemy, physicians took account of aethereal forces, and the Moon with its cycles retained a role in the humoural model. Reverend Harley, in his compendium of moon lore, quoted the bleeding strategy of French court physician and botanist La Martinière:

> This lunar planet is damp of itself, but, by the radiation of the sun, is of various temperaments, as follows: in its first quadrant it is warm and damp, at which time it is good to let the blood of sanguine persons; in its second it is warm and dry, at which time it is good to bleed the choleric; in its third quadrant it is cold and moist, and phlegmatic people may be bled; and in its fourth it is cold and dry, at which time it is well to bleed the melancholic.[20]

Phlebotomy was thus administered as prophylaxis to lunar excitation. Francis Bacon attributed much power to the Moon. As bodily humours rose and fell to a lunar regularity, he advised people with moist brains to take *Lignus aloe*, rosemary or frankincense at full moon. In his *Natural History* he claimed that infants born at full moon would grow sturdier than those delivered on the wane.

17   Chapman A (1979): 'Astrological medicine'. In *Health, Medicine and Mortality in the Sixteenth Century* (ed. C Webster), 275–300.

18   Quoted in Hone (1978), p294.

19   Webster C (1979): 'Alchemical and Paracelsian medicine'. In *Health, Medicine and Mortality in the Sixteenth Century* (ed. C Webster), 301–334, p314.

20   Quoted in Harley T (1885): *Moon Lore*. London: Swan Sonnenschein, Le Bas & Lowry, p196.

Meanwhile the mystical luminary continued to exercise the popular imagination, and its alleged ability to unhinge minds was perpetuated by novelists and playwrights. John Milton referred to 'moonstruck madness' in *Paradise Lost*. A character of T Adams, another English writer of the seventeenth century, had a 'moonsick head'. References appeared throughout Shakespeare's dramas: there were 'lunes' (mad fits of distraction) in *The Winter's Tale*, and this intriguing passage in *Othello*:[21]

> It is the very error of the moon
> She comes more nearer earth
> than she was wont
> And makes men mad.

21   William Shakespeare (1604/1996). *Othello*. Act V, scene II. *Complete Works of William Shakespeare*. Wordsworth.

Three

Lunacy in the Age of Reason

When the moon's in the full, then wit's in the wane.

The Witch of Edmonton (Dekker, Ford and Rowley, 1658)

While supernatural beliefs prevailed in the common people, there was a marked decline in magic and demonology within educated circles in the late seventeenth century, hastened by scientific discoveries and the ascent of reason. Scholarly ways of knowing the world diverged into two opposing standpoints. First, there was empiricism, credited to Francis Bacon, a prominent administrator of the English Crown. Knowledge, according to Bacon, emanated from first-hand experience, not from deferring to the texts of antiquity. He elevated utility over theoretical debate, and presented a manifesto of cumulative fact drawn from multiple observations and observers, to discover and exploit the laws of nature to the benefit of the kingdom and its subjects. This contrasted with the rationalism of René Descartes (1596–1650), in whose treatise *Discours de la Methode, pour bien conduire la Raison et chercher la Vérité dans les Sciences* experiment was always to be preceded by argument. Descartes looked beyond mathematics and logic in his pursuit of certainty, which could never be reached through our flawed sensory capacity, but relied on reason. In proposing rules for generating knowledge, both Bacon and Descartes made a significant contribution to scientific progress.

Descartes addressed himself to the epistemological challenge of understanding human thought and behaviour. The physical world had properties limited to size, form and motion, and was governed by mathematical laws; animals were mere automata, as assemblies of tissue with no inherent purpose beyond survival. Human beings, however, rose above bodily functions to act rationally: it was the soul set man apart from beast. Anticipatory truth was demonstrated by the dictum *cogito, ergo sum*: awareness of self was inherent. Descartes speculated interaction of mind and matter at the pineal gland, where the 'vital energy' of the soul converted into physical action. In the Cartesian dualism of perception and cognition, vision involved sensory mechanics alone, but interpreting an image was a rational process. Qualities such as colour and taste did not exist physically, but only in the mind.

The most influential thinker of his time, Descartes devised a credible model of the cosmos. Abhorring a vacuum, he claimed that the celestial bodies moved in swirling vortices, surrounded not by space but immersed in a whirlpool of ether. Such theory was blown away by the outstanding figure of the Scientific Enlightenment, Isaac Newton (1643–1727). As an early sign of his genius, Newton had devised the reflecting telescope, its curved mirror in place of refractory lens overcoming the problem of light distortion. Optics was Newton's forte before he turned to the conundra of motion and gravity. Without sufficient friction to check their trajectories, Newton wondered why the planets did not move in a straight line through space: what maintained their elliptical orbits? It was the motion of the Moon around Earth on which he developed his hypothesis. From the estimated circumference of Earth, and the distance from its satellite, Newton confirmed his putative law of universal gravitation, as described in his *Philosophie Naturalis Principia Mathematica*: 'Every particle of matter in the universe attracts every other particle with a force varying inversely as the square of the distance between them and directly as the product of the masses of the two particles.'[1]

Thus the same force by which the legendary apple plummeted from a branch in a Lincolnshire garden governed how the celestial bodies move in space and time. Lunar regulation of tides was confirmed, although here imagination had preceded science; Shakespeare had referred to the Moon as 'governess of floods' in *Midsummer Night's Dream*. Newton acknowledged his scientific predecessors thus: 'If I have seen further than others, it was because I stood upon the shoulders of giants.' He owed much to Dutch astronomer Christiaan Huygens (1629–1695) for his formulae for centrifugal force, which provided the antagonist of gravity in maintaining planets in their orbits.[2] He was also indebted to Kepler and Galileo, who had both mistakenly regarded gravity as a magnetic force, undoubtedly influenced by William Gilbert's description of Earth as a giant lodestone. The laws of motion and universal gravitation forged an important bond between terrestrial and celestial phenomena: as envisaged by Plato, the workings of the universe could be expressed as mathematical equations.

The advance of science in western culture was demonstrated by the inauguration in 1662 of the Royal Society for the Advancement of Experimental Philosophy in London; and four years later the *Académie Royale des Sciences* in Paris, with Huygens as its most illustrious founding member.

---

1   Published 1685-1687; quoted in Hone (1978), pp294-295.
2   For his work on astronomy the great Dutch scientist is honoured by the tallest peak on the Moon, Mons Huygens in the Apennines, at 15,000 feet.

Paris pursued the physico-mathematics of Descartes; London the Baconian manifesto of practical empiricism. The Moon drew much interest in these academic circles, not only in selenography, but also in relation to the most important scientific problem of the time: measurement of longitude at sea. This was the 'age of sail', when nations were competing for mercantile supremacy. A multitude of sailors perished in ships wrecked off the coast or lost without trace due to an inability to determine position in the vast, inhospitable oceans. The compass, as transpired in the transatlantic voyages of Columbus, was unreliable due to magnetic variations, as well as a wildly swinging needle. Precise latitudinal and longitudinal coordinates could be obtained through telescopic observation of the moons of Jupiter, but this required a steady instrument, and was impracticable at sea. A Royal Commission was established by Charles II to resolve the navigational problem. The lunar distances method, in which longitude was calculated from the angle between the Moon and another celestial body, was unreliable due to perturbations of the lunar course. Its refinement occupied the first Astronomer Royal John Flamsteed for forty years at the new observatory of Greenwich, and the Moon remained the guide to longitude until well into the nineteenth century.[3]

From a Christian perspective, the Moon and planets were not dislodged from their heavenly status, but accommodation of advances in astronomy was necessary to avert a widening gap between faith and reason. Descartes had presented a rational argument for the existence of a Supreme Being, while compatriot and fellow mathematician Blaise Pascal (1623–1663) asserted that proof of God was beyond our capacities of perception and comprehension (Pascal is renowned for his wager, whereby the most rational position is to believe in God, because for the gambler it minimises losses should such belief transpire as erroneous, with potentially infinite reward). In most countries it remained dangerous to express heretical ideas, but from the tolerant atmosphere of Holland arose a radical reinterpretation of divinity. Benedictus de Spinoza (1632–1677) claimed that God and Universe were one, an infinite existence beyond anthropic concern, and in his deterministic view of nature, the free will afforded by Christian faith was an illusion. For this transgression, Spinoza was excommunicated by the Amsterdam Jewry. Philosophical conjecture such as pantheism could be dismissed, but as more mysteries of nature were unravelled, religious truth was threatened. Fortunately Newton was

---

3   The lunar distances method was superseded by the marine chronometer. In 1714 the British government, anxious to prevent further tragedies at sea, offered a £20,000 prize to anyone who could overcome an obstacle thought insurmountable by Newton. Finally, a self-educated Yorkshire carpenter, John Harrison (1693-1776) produced the clock that allowed sailors to know their exact point in longitude, although this expensive device did not become widely used until a hundred years later.

a committed believer who attributed his universal laws to Providence, and he occupied an influential position as president of the Royal Society from 1702 until his death in 1727. Theologians argued that science revealed, but could not ultimately explain. Astronomers were simply illuminating the magnificence of divine creation, as reflected in this seventeenth century hymn by Joseph Addison:[4]

> The spacious firmament on high,
> With all the blue ethereal sky,
> And spangled heavens, a shining frame,
> Their great Original proclaim.
> The unwearied sun from day to day
> Does his Creator's power display,
> And publishes to every land
> The works of an almighty hand.

The seventeenth century brought tremendous progress in anatomy and physiology, and the traditional humoural system began to subside under a volley of contrary evidence from surgical experience. Although the Church had generally opposed dissection, dispensations were issued periodically for medical research and teaching.[5] Demonstrations on criminal cadavers began as a teaching method in Bologna around 1300, and the first anatomical textbook based on dissection was written by Mondino de'Leuzzi (1275–1326). Operations entailed running commentary by a medical professor while lower-status surgeons did the dirty work. This was the convention until Andreas Vesalius (1514–1564), professor of surgery and anatomy at Padua (then the leading medical school in Europe), grasped the scalpel. In 1543 Vesalius produced his seminal and intricately illustrated work *The Fabric of the Human Body*, which mostly supported classic anatomical knowledge, but corrected some major errors, reverently attributed to Galen being restricted to examining the Barbary ape. The detailed images by anatomical artist Leonardo da Vinci (1452–1519), informed by human dissection, had also strayed from medical theory. In the mid-seventeenth century, Descartes produced what is considered the first textbook on human physiology; his *Treatise on Man* was a theoretical rather than observational work, but its importance was in its depiction of the human body as a machine.

The most significant breakthrough in physiology was in 1628, when William Harvey (1578–1657) explained the hydrostatic circulatory system on which life depended. Galen had described the veins and arteries as separate entities, with arterial blood carrying heat and *pneuma* from the heart,

---

4   Quoted in Patey EH (1978): *All in Good Faith*. Oxford: Mowbrays, p31.
5   Park K (2009): 'Myth 5: That the medieval church prohibited human dissection'. In *Galileo goes to Jail and Other Myths about Science and Religion* (ed. RL Numbers). New York: Harvard University Press.

and venous blood delivering nutrients from the liver. In his *Exertatio Anatomica de Motu Cordis at Sanguinis in Animalibus (Essay on the Anatomy of the Heart and Blood of Animals)*, Harvey refuted the hepatic source and the consumption of blood by tissues, and showed that the heart is not a repository but a pump, with all blood passing through the lungs. Initially, the Parisian medical establishment continued teaching Galen, but Harvey's discovery was supported by the microscopic investigations of Marcello Malpighi (1628–1694) of Bologna, who found the capillary link between the blood vessels going to and from the heart.

The use of lens to reveal the minute workings of the body was another scientific odyssey that began in the Netherlands. Like other linen merchants, Anton von Leeuwenhoek (1632–1723) had been using a glass lens to check consistencies of thread, but his curiosity led to wider adventures in the miniature world. Investigating the constituents of water, blood and semen, he observed tiny units of life that he thought were tiny versions of animals, or 'animalcules'. Unwittingly, this amateur scientist had discovered the cell.[6] Such endeavour cemented medicine into the realm of science. Medical students flocked to Leyden, where the inspirational teacher Herman Boerhaave (1668–1738) demonstrated the microscopic study of tissue.

In the Cartesian-inspired Age of Reason, madness, as an affectation of the soul rather than of the body, was construed by some scholars not as illness but as folly. According to Michel Foucault in his historical account, *Madness and Civilisation*, this was the 'classical period', when reason was the defining feature of humanity. Unbridled passions were a threat to civil order, and began to attract administrative interventions, such as the 'Ship of Fools' sailing up and down the Rhine. Public fascination in the spectre of madness was illustrated by the vast numbers attracted to the Bethlem Hospital in London, where visitors, for a charge of one penny, could stare at the wretched inmates and goad them into tantrums. At a time when madness was yet to be colonised by medicine, the insane were readily reduced to the status of brutes. Meanwhile, physicians of Galenic persuasion continued to attribute mental disturbance to bodily dysfunction. The spleen was blamed for melancholia, insanity and epilepsy, while hysteria, as the name suggests, was associated with the uterus.

New perspectives on mind and madness were offered by British empiricist philosophers. Taking materialism to the extreme, Thomas Hobbes (1588–1679) described mental activity as merely particles of the brain in motion. There was also the *tabula rasa* of John Locke, each person's character and intellect being formed purely by experience. Locke was a former student of Thomas Willis, who initiated systematic investigation of the brain. The organ had been believed to be of fluid consistency, as indicated

---

6   Much later, in 1838, Theodor Schwann identified this structure as the basic unit of all living matter.

by the grey mush leaking from the skulls of battle casualties, but Willis differentiated a firm structure of brain stem, medulla and fissures. He was first to describe the nerves as solid tissue, and coined the term 'neurology'. Knowledge of the nervous system remained primitive, but Willis' work was instrumental in confirming the brain as the centre of sensation and cognition. Locke, whom Voltaire dubbed 'anatomist of the soul', described madness as a disease of ideas. In his *Essay on Human Understanding* of 1690, he distinguished disturbance of imagination caused by unruly passions (as often occurred in people of artistic talent) from loss of reason, the latter being the defining feature of insanity.

Madness was thus caught in a no-man's land between mind and matter. Discussing the reciprocal action of body and soul in disease, Georg Ernst von Stahl (1660–1734), professor of medicine at Halle, asserted that medicine should be concerned with both. For von Stahl, the body was subject to higher laws than those of mechanics and chemical process, all human activity depending on a vital spirit, which he named 'anima'. This integrative concept followed the monism of Spinoza, whereby body and mind were not separate entities in interaction, but different attributes of the same being. This early version of psychosomatic theory provided a philosophical basis for medical interest in madness. However, with physicalism driving the advance of medical knowledge, mind was subordinated to brain. A physiological concepualisation of insanity gained ground, reviving the teachings of Hippocrates, who had regarded insanity as corporeal disease.

With no bodily seat of madness found, new theories on insanity overlapped with older ideas. Just as alchemy gradually transformed into chemistry, humoural medicine did not suddenly disappear on the discovery of the circulatory system. Abstract essences had begun to dissolve into a mechanistic model of particles and pipelines, but prominent physicians maintained aspects of the classical system; Boerhaave, for example, continued to attribute melancholia to excesses of black bile. His students William Cullen and John Pringle, who helped found the medical schools of Glasgow and Edinburgh, reinforced humoural concepts well into the eighteenth century. English physician Sir Richard Blackmore maintained the aetiological focus on the spleen in his *Treatise of the Spleen and Vapours* of 1725. Just as terms such as 'phlegmatic' outlived humoural medicine, the concept of passions lingered in medical theories of mental disturbance. Melancholia and mania, if they became fixed, might not only impair the soul but also cause chronic laxity and density of brain fibres, thus destroying the individual's connection with reality.

As the eighteenth century progressed, there was a tendency for writers to accept the brain and nerves as the location of madness. Humoural theory was replaced by a speculative mechanical model, akin to the cardiovascular system. Unruly motion of nervous fluid was thought to result from all kinds of provocative factors, including the weather, bad air, intemperance and an overactive imagination, as described in *The English Malady*, the classic treatise on madness by George Cheyne (1673–1743). [7] However, severe forms of mental derangement were likely to be seen as inherent fault in the individual, independent of exciting cause. In insanity proper, environmental factors were considered of less import. Although it was widely believed that the Moon could affect mental states, its presumed causative powers were receding.

Gravity and the mind

Abandonment of superstition by the ruling class was associated with growing authority of disciplines such as medicine, in which empiricism had brought great progress. Yet there was much to be learned about the biochemical processes of the body; the invisible workings of the brain were uncharted territory, and the pharmacopoeia was confined to rudimentary concoctions (a paucity that would continue until the emergence of industrial chemistry in the mid-nineteenth century). While astrology had been banished, old ideas about cosmic forces on health were revived by Newtonian physics. Lunar regulation of tidal rhythms, confirmed in Newton's *Principia*, stimulated medical interest in gravity. Botanist Nehemiah Grew (1641–1712), in his *Cosmologica Sacra* of 1701, postulated that both Sun and Moon exerted a gravitational force on bodily fluids, most visibly manifest in menstruation, epilepsy and lunacy. The same principle was applied to the fluid of the nervous system by Richard Mead (1673–1754), an acquaintance of Newton, and physician to King George II. He stated that females were more susceptible to mental disturbance at certain phases of the Moon due to its regulation of menstrual cycles. According to Mead, the conditions that tended to follow lunar cycles were nephritis, ulcers, asthma, hysteria and epilepsy. In his *Treatise Concerning the Influence of the Sun and Moon upon Human Bodies*, Mead reflected on a recurring mental aberration:

> When I was physician to St Thomas's hospital during the time of Queen Anne's wars with France, several of the sailors of our fleets were brought thither, and put under my care for distemper: most of whom were new men, who had contacted the disease by frights, either

7   Cheyne G (1734): *The English Malady, or a Treatise on Nervous Diseases of All Kinds.* London: Strahan & Leake. The concept of nervous fluid lingered despite no proof of its existence.

in sea-engagements, or in storms. But the Moon's influence was so visible on the generality of them at the new and the full, that I have often predicted the times of the fits with tolerable certainty.[8]

Mead reported similar observations by fellow physicians, such as William Pitcairne (1711–1791), reputed botanist and physician at St Bartholomew's Hospital in London. Mead believed that lunar influence peaked at perigee and apogee.

The link between mind and cosmos was resurrected by the late eighteenth century advent of mesmerism. In a renewal of vitalism, Franz Anton Mesmer (1733–1815) believed in a pervasive force that maintained cosmic harmony and affected all life on Earth. In his 1766 doctoral thesis *Physico-medica de Planetarium Influxa*, Mesmer applied the Newtonian concept of imponderable fluids to physiology. He had read the treatise *De Medicina Magnetica* by English physician William Maxwell (1581–1641), which had propounded the theory of a vital spirit transmittable through touch or proximity, thus integrating material and spiritual life. The mid to late eighteenth century was a time of important discoveries in the invisible forces of electricity and magnetism. The Leyden jar, a basic electrical capacitator that issued a mild shock, was a drawing room entertainment. Benjamin Franklin (1706-1790) became a scientific celebrity after his experiments with a kite proved that lightning was an electrical phenomenon, leading to his invention of the lightning rod. Commercial production of magnets as scientific equipment had begun in the 1740s.

Mesmer postulated a universal magnetic fluid permeating all inanimate and organic bodies, in which interruptions of flow would account for various maladies. While practising medicine in Vienna, he became acquainted with English astrologer and Jesuit priest Maximilian Hell, who claimed to have cured several cases of abdominal cramp with a magnet. Medical application of magnets had originated in the Orient, and featured in the practice of Paracelsus, but Mesmer was first to present a theoretical rationale. Experimenting with Hell's magnets, Mesmer speculated that the apparent therapeutic benefits derived from manipulation of ethereal motions, analogous to lunar magnetic pull on the oceans. The treatment stimulated convulsive muscular twitching and a trance-like state. Soon, he found that similar effects were achieved by stroking affected parts with his bare hands, which he attributed to the flow of his own healthy magnetism. Startling cures were announced, particularly in nervous disorders.

On publishing his findings in 1775 Mesmer received much hostility from the Viennese medical circle, but Louis XVI invited him to Paris, where he

---

8   Mead R (1746): 'Treatise concerning the influence of the Sun and Moon upon human bodies, and the diseases thereby produced'. In *The Medical Works of Richard Mead*. Dublin: Thomas Ewing, p113-156.

became an overnight sensation. Such was demand that Mesmer initiated group therapy using a circular tub filled with magnetic filings, with multiple handles so that up to thirty patients could engage simultaneously with the flow of magnetism. Mesmer imperiously circulated the group in his silk robes, touching patients with his wand to hasten the effect, akin to the 'King's Touch' (a popular belief in seventeenth century France and England of the divine powers of monarchs to cure disease by contact). After the Academy of Sciences snubbed his invitation to witness his treatment, he threatened to leave Paris, but Queen Marie Antoinette paid him to stay, and his appointments in the parlours of the noblesse resumed.

Accusations of quackery were rife in eighteenth century medicine, and in 1784 King Louis XVI appointed a committee enquiring into the practice, comprising four members of the Parisian Society of Medicine and five men of the *Académie Royale des Sciences*. Among the esteemed scientists was Antoine-Laurent Lavoisier, best known for his work in chemistry and human respiration, and chairing the committee was American ambassador and grandee of scientific enquiry, Benjamin Franklin. Mesmer was confident in his curative powers, but the investigators were not interested in the beliefs of patients or doctors, focusing only on physical proof of animal magnetism. They uncovered several falsehoods; for example, a patient who had allegedly recovered after contact with a 'magnetised' tree had actually clasped a nearby trunk instead. It transpired that other cures had been achieved when patients had actually held inert lead discs rather than magnetic zinc. The report found no evidence of electrical or magnetic activity, and dismissed the process as imaginary. They concluded: '*L'imagination fait tout; le magnétisme nul.*'[9]

The scientific experts had not seen the wood for the trees. Mesmerism thrived long after Mesmer's death, and while exploited by charlatans, it was practised at reputable clinics for all kinds of physical ailments. In his book *Neurypnology* of 1843, Manchester surgeon James Braid coined the term 'hypnosis' (from the Greek meaning 'sleep') for the dreamlike state produced by mesmerism. Its use in operative surgery continued until the arrival of chemical anaethesia in the 1850s.[10] As for the authority of the Academy, this was the body that had endorsed Thomas Jefferson's rejection of the seemingly fantastical idea that rocks, or meterorites, could fall from the sky.

9   Quoted in Szasz T (2007): *Cure and Coercion*. Piscataway, NJ: Transaction.
10   Marcuse FL (1959): *Hypnosis: Fact and Fiction*. Harmondsworth: Penguin.

Scientism and the evaporation of spirits

Just as alchemy was replaced by chemistry, the animal magnetism contro-versy illustrated the progress in medicine from an abstract 'art of healing' to a scrutinised body of knowledge. The late eighteenth century was the zenith of scientific materialism, which had inspired Utopian ideals of human mastery of nature. Facts were there to be discovered. Faith and supernaturalism was undermined by arch empiricist David Hume (1711–1776). Dismissing abstract ideas not conducive to verification or mathematical measurement, Hume argued that metaphysics should be 'committed to the flames, for it can contain nothing but sophistry and illu-sion'.[11] Hume argued that there could be no certainty in scientific laws, because all that could be known was from observation, and causal rela-tionships are a product of the mind; instead, science proceeds as 'miti-gated scepticism'.

Bold empiricism was restrained by the brilliant mind of Königsberg, Immanuel Kant (1724–1804). In his seminal *Kritik der reinen Vernunft (Cri-tique of Pure Reason)* of 1871, Kant argued that without reason, observation was mere perception, and thus subjective. Fact and theory in science pro-ceed like left and right feet: neither can go more than one step ahead of the other.[12] Making sense of the world, according to Kant, relies on innate cat-egories of interpretation. Three-dimensional space, and the relationship between cause and effect, are examples of a programmed framework of comprehension. As we are limited to our cognitive and sensory tools for processing information, we cannot know reality: the universe is infinite, but perceptual capacity finite. With his profound view of metaphysics, Kant hammered the final nail in the coffin of teleology in the realm of sci-ence. Kantian agnosticism left the door ajar for a supreme being, but faith occupied a transcendental domain beyond the reach of science.

When Kant first put pen to paper, the accepted age of the universe remained on a Biblical scale. Based on the lifespan of patriarchs of the Old Testament, in 1620 Archbishop Ussher of Armagh had timed genesis at

---

11 Quoted in Blackburn S (1994): *The Oxford Dictionary of Philosophy*. Oxford: Oxford University Press, p240.

12 This analogy borrowed from J Bronowski (1951): *The Common Sense of Science*. London: Heinemann.

nightfall on 23rd October 4004 BC. From patterns of geological erosion, Edmund Halley (1656–1742), who was immortalised by the correctly predicted return of a comet sixteen years after his death, extended the estimated age to over six thousand years BC. By the eighteenth century, the fossil finds of paleontologists raised serious doubts about such recency, and literal interpretation of Scripture was untenable. In 1750 Thomas Wright had observed that the Milky Way was an enormous disc, and powerful telescopes revealed that many distant nebulae were similarly shaped. This suggested to Kant an infinite number of galaxies, all revolving around an unknown point. He surmised that the Universe began as nebula of randomly colliding molecules, producing a condensing mass of gas and stars, set into eternal rotation by the force of collision. Kant's speculative cosmogony restricted the need for a prime mover to the first day of Creation.

The primal nebula idea was placed on a firmer footing by the French astronomer Pierre Simon de Laplace, whose *Mécanique Céleste*, published in five volumes from 1799 to 1825, developed Newton's laws into a comprehensive mathematical model to explain all known celestial peturbations. Laplace noted four common features of the planets: they revolve in the same direction, rotate in the same direction; move on the same plane, and have almost circular ellipses. He speculated that as a primal nebula cooled, its ellipse became stretched by centrifugal force, eventually producing a disc form. Outer rings then broke free from the primeval star, spinning faster under centrifugal force until they crystallised into spheres. In just two centuries, our knowledge of the cosmos had advanced from deciphering the orbits of the Moon and planets, to answering major questions about the universe. The evolution of the stars was explained, and no divine levers were required in a mechanical system of infinite galaxies. Fundamentally, the Kant–Laplace model prevails to this day.

In the dizzy heights of scientific materialism it was believed that everything in the physical universe would eventually yield to deterministic law. Investigating the underlying forces of nature required the specialist, armed with sophisticated equipment, drilling deeper into the mineshaft of his subject without gazing across the wider terrain. The goal of natural philosophy had thus shifted from what Thomas Aquinas referred to as 'the slenderest knowledge that may be obtained of the highest things'to precise knowledge of the specific.[13] Nature was a machine to be dismantled, made predictable, and ultimately controlled. The status of traditional truth was undermined: either an idea must be amenable to scientific enquiry, or it must remain in the realm of the spiritual or metaphysical. Enduring beliefs such as that of lunar influence on mind or body, not only had to be logical (for example, based on the theory of gravity), but also ver-

---

13   Quoted in Schumacher EF (1977): *A Guide for the Perplexed*. London: Abacus, p65.

ified by systematic observation. However, just as the telescope was blind to cosmic forces, the microscope could not discern the invisible workings of the human mind. Medicine had embraced an *a posteriori* epistemology of observable signs and symptoms, and as nascent specialisms emerged, holistic concepts of a life force disappeared from medical discourse. The noble art had evolved from the landscape artists of Paracelsan astro-medicine to the intricate detail of the miniaturist. In its fascination with the organism, no longer would medicine consult the moon and stars. An epitaph for the polymath was inscribed by Arthur Koestler:[14]

> The *uomo universale* of the Renaissance, who was artist and craftsman, philosopher and inventor, humanist and scientist, astronomer and monk, all in one, split up into his component parts. Art lost its mythical, science its mystical inspiration; man became again deaf to the harmony of the spheres.

14   Koestler A (1964): *The Sleepwalkers: A History of Man's Changing Vision of the Universe.* Harmondsworth: Penguin, p549-550.

Four

Eclipsed by mental science

Madness has transcended the ages as a pained or chaotic expression of the human condition, but only in the last two hundred years did its study and treatment emerge as a specialist discipline. Over millennia the mad had drawn curiosity and fear, their fate fluctuating between charity and persecution. In the patchwork of hamlets and market towns in pre-industrial Britain and western Europe, parishes consumed their own smoke; mentally unsound individuals, popularly depicted as the 'village idiot', were often beneficiaries of informal social services. Others of wandering minds took to a wayfaring existence, joining the circus of itinerant vagrants reliant on alms, petty wages and whatever opportunities came their way. Monastic sanctuaries appeared sporadically, notably Bethlem Hospital in London and at Gheel in Belgium, but these were few and far between. As urbanisation proceeded, the city became a magnet for tortured souls. In Britain, some subscription-funded infirmaries emerging in provincial towns in the eighteenth century included a lunatic annex, but the insane were more likely to be held in penal establishments or placed at the mercy of the burgeoning madhouse trade, where pecuniary gain of unscrupulous proprietors was maximised by prolonged incarceration. The plight of the mad was brought to public attention, firstly by the harsh treatment meted to King George III in his episodes of derangement, and by a series of scandals exposing dreadful conditions in private madhouses. Eventually, campaigners succeeded in raising state intervention, materialising in a regulated system of public lunatic asylums.

The legal category of lunacy

Affecting the capacity of the individual, madness had become a matter of legal concern. In English law a distinction was made between those with congenital mental defect (then labelled 'idiots'), and the insane. Insanity excluded milder forms of mental disorder such as melancholia, where the cognitive faculties were generally retained. For the judiciary, the definition related to reason rather than clinical characteristics. Sir Edward Coke (1552–1634) had devised four categories: idiots; persons who had lost their minds through sickness, grief or accident; self-inflicted insanity as in drunkards; and lunatics. The latter term was not synonymous with madness, but was a recurring affliction with lucid intervals. In the first known book devoted to English law on madness, written for a lay audience by John Brydall in 1700, the legal status *non compos mentis* comprised three categories: 'natural fools' (those born with mental defect); 'mad-folk' (those who had lost their mental faculties), and 'lunatick persons'.[1] The first statutory provision in England specifically for the mentally disturbed was the Vagrancy Act of 1744, previous acts having treated the insane no differently from vagbonds. The Act encompassed both the permanently and monthly insane:

> It shall and may be lawful for any two or more Justices of the Peace where such lunatic or mad person shall be found, by warrant under their hands and seals, directed to the constables, churchwardens and overseers of the poor of such Parish, Town or Place, to cause such persons to be apprehended and kept safely locked up in some secure place as such Justices shall appoint; and (if such Justices find it necessary) to be there chained.[2]

The notion of lunar influence was reinforced in the conceptualisation of madness by Lord Chief Justice Sir Matthew Hale (1609–1676), whose *History of Pleas of the Crown*, published sixty years after his death, described 'permanent' and 'interpolating' dementia. He explained:

> ... the latter is that which is usually called lunacy, for the moon hath a great influence in all diseases of the brain, especially in this kind of dementia; such persons commonly in the full and change of the moon, especially about the equinoxes and summer solstice, are usually at the height of their distemper.[3]

Hale was writing on criminal law, but his differentiation of permanent and episodic was important in civil law, as lunatics fluctuated in ability to understand their affairs. The lunatic label was not always used in eighteenth century medical texts, some physicians preferring the overarching term 'insanity' for the delusional forms of mental disorder, whether acute, recurring or chronic. By contrast, English statutes began to refer to 'lunatics' generically for the status *non compos mentis*. In his celebrated work

1   Hunter and Macalpine (1963).
2   Quoted in Skultans V (1979): *English Madness: Ideas on Insanity 1580-1890*. London: Routledge & Kegan Paul, p106.
3   Quoted in Hale M (1736): *History of the Pleas of the Crown*. London: E & R Nutt and R Gosling, p30.

Commentaries on the Laws of England of 1765–1769, eminent English judge Sir William Blackstone acknowledged the broadening definition, but reinforced the meaning of true lunacy:

> A lunatic, or non compos mentis, is one who hath had understanding, but by disease, grief or other accident hath lost the use of his reason. A lunatic is properly one that hath lucid intervals; sometimes enjoying his senses and sometimes not and that frequently depending upon the changes of the moon.[4]

The aetiology of madness was not a legal concern, but how were jurists informed on this periodical affliction somehow influenced by the Moon? Medical testimony was not generally sought in English courts until the nineteenth century, and no judge was likely to deal with many cases of the intermittent form of madness. Historians have suggested that Blackstone's conception would have related to manic-depressive conditions, but some presentations of epilepsy would also have fitted his criteria of regular patterns of irrationality and lucid intervals.

Although epilepsy was considered by many physicians to be a natural disease, in the seventeenth century Georg Stahl had explained seizures as an expression of emotional disturbance, and Thomas Willis had attributed mild convulsions to psychogenic cause. Indeed Willis, who saw epilepsy as a sign of *incubus*, had considered hysteria not as a uterine condition but as a convulsive disorder. The Graeco-Roman link between epilepsy and hysteria was revived, with George Cheyne seeing no basic difference between epilepsy and hysteria in his noted work *The English Malady* of 1733. Seizures were thus regarded as manifestations of mental disorder, and Blackstone may have been guided by the reports of distinguished physician Richard Mead of lunar regulation. However, Swiss physician Simon André Tissot (1728–1797), in his seminal *Traité de l'Épilepsie* in 1770, rejected the long established link between the Moon and epilepsy, arguing that monthly periodicity did not infer causal influence.

Throughout the British Empire, where care and control of all mentally incapacitated persons was covered by 'lunacy' laws, the concept of lunar influence was preserved by institutionalised misnomer. Although remnants of the Lunacy Act of 1890 remained in force in Britain until the beginning of the 1960s, this was an artefact. Nineteenth century jurisprudence was sceptical of the concept, as illustrated by the case of Charles Hyde, a labourer who pleaded that his awful crimes were provoked by the phases of the Moon. His defence fell on deaf ears and he was jailed, but he inspired the 1886 novel by Robert Louis Stevenson: *Doctor Jekyll and Mister Hyde*.

---

4   Blackstone W (1765): *Commentaries on the Laws of England*. Oxford: Clarendon Press, p293.

Birth of the asylum

An imposing Gothic edifice is the indelible image of the asylum. To some people, those brick towers looming on the horizon stirred memories of oppression; to others, a sad demise of a refuge from an uncaring society. The archipelago of mental institutions in the countryside was the birthplace of psychiatry, the branch of medicine concerned with the diagnosis and treatment of mental illness. Two parallel developments share primacy in the asylum movement. Of profound influence in Britain was The Retreat near York, a philanthropic establishment opened in 1796 by tea and coffee merchant William Tuke (1732–1822) and family, who were devout Quakers. Applying the original concept of asylum as a temporary respite from life's distress, The Retreat was characterised by a humane regime whereby patients were coaxed back to sanity in a dignified *milieu* of fresh air, wholesome diet and productive occupation. Reputedly even the most frenzied individuals were restored to reason and enabled to resume their roles in the community. While the Tukes devised a moral form of rehabilitation, Paris is credited with the beginnings of specialised medical treatment of the insane.

In 1794 Philippe Pinel (1745–1826) became superintendent at the Bicêtre institution, which originated in the Hôpital Général network founded in 1657 by the Parisian authorities. This was not a hospital in the medical sense, but housed various social deviants sent by judicial order. By the 1790s both the Bicêtre and La Salpêtrière premises had become depositories for the insane, where Pinel found the miserable inmates suffering in squalor and physical restraint. Rejecting the nihilistic view of madness as incurable, he transformed the regime. His first subject of liberation was an old English captain, who had been incarcerated for forty years, and yet had managed to kill an attendant with a blow from his manacles. Talking to this refractory inmate in his cell, Pinel merely asked for gentlemanly behaviour in return for removing the irons, and the old sailor kept his promise. In his widely translated *Traité Médico-philosophique sur l'Aliénation Mentale, ou la Manie*, first published in 1801, he declared: 'How necessary it is, in order to forestall hypochondria, melancholia, or mania to follow the immutable laws of morality'.[5] For Pinel, moral management was a means of exerting discipline on unstable emotions, a medical orien-

5   Pinel P (1801): *Traité Médico-philosophique sur l'Aliénation Mentale*. Paris: Antoine Brosson, p238–239.

tation unlike the egalitarian spirit of the Tukes. Semantic differences aside, the common theme was the primacy of care over control. Moral management was espoused as the model for lunatic asylums throughout the western world.

The fact that the system of pauper lunatic asylums and industrial revolution developed most rapidly in Britain was no coincidence. Sprawling conurbations were built around manufacturing hubs, where reliance on cheap labour generated a vast working class. The privations of grim factory towns spawned multitudes of social casualties. As traditional bonds were shattered by rapid social change, economically inactive adults became a burden on relatives. Order among the unruly and intemperate masses was instilled through a combination of philanthropy and authoritarian measures. While evangelical activists urged institutional provision to rescue the poor from a life of vice and despair, from the utilitarian perspective it served society through the principle of the greater good for the greater number. Philosopher-jurist Jeremy Bentham (1748–1832) designed the 'panopticon', a model institution for large numbers of inmates, which maximised surveillance and efficiency. This archetype was followed in the design of prisons, but was generally considered inappropriate for the supposedly therapeutic environment of the asylum.

Meanwhile another important social institution, the workhouse, proliferated in the early nineteenth century, and provided a haven for lunatics washed up alongside the indigent and invalid in a general tide of destitution. Here, inmate labour served both moral and economic purpose, being considered the route to salvation, while enabling the institution to pay its way, thus reducing the burden on ratepayers. Unpredictable and disruptive to the strict regime, mentally disturbed inmates were treated harshly by workhouse masters, and were typically confined in the darkest and dingiest corners of these Spartan structures. The campaign for appropriate provision for the insane continued, and county authorities in Britain that had dragged their heels on building a lunatic asylum, mainly due to expense, were eventually compelled by the 1845 Lunatic Asylums Act.

The asylums were designed to provide environmental attributes akin to The Retreat, with south-facing layouts maximising fresh air and sunlight, surrounded by acres of fertile land. Palatial façades, an expression of civic pride, masked the austerity of the interior, but for the majority of pauper inmates, conditions were superior to the harsh lives left behind at the asylum gates. However, the initially small county asylums rapidly exceeded capacity. As sociologist Andrew Scull argued in *Museums of Madness*, the expanding provision of lunatic asylums encouraged a broadening definition of insanity.[6] As receptacles not only for the acutely

6   Scull AT (1979): *Museums of Madness: the Social Organization of Insanity in 19th Century England*. London: Allen Lane.

mad but also for intractable social problems, asylums grew into vast human warehouses, and by mid-century the average size in England reached three hundred beds. To alleviate overcrowding, populous counties eventually resorted to building second asylums. In 1851 the Middlesex authority opened the thousand-bed Colney Hatch Asylum for the east of the county, but within a few years demand outstripped supply, necessitating new blocks of hundreds more beds before the decade was out. Towards the end of the century additional asylums for the urban catchments of Lancashire, Yorkshire and London were being built for over two thousand inmates. State asylums in America were larger still, some extending beyond four thousand beds, in enormous multi-storey blocks. Individual attention was inevitably neglected, as inmates were herded around by a small uneducated band of attendants, the jangle of keys echoing along gloomy corridors. In this degrading environment, the proportion of 'cures' declined.

The birth of the asylum has attracted wide scholarly interest, with sociological revisions of history challenging the conventional version of the rescue of the insane by medical heroics. In Scull's aforementioned polemic, the asylum programme was a segregative sanction to coerce the labour market into conformity; *avant garde* philosopher Michel Foucault rejected progressive assumptions, claiming that rather than liberating the mad, the asylum functioned as an instrument of capitalist discipline beneath a veneer of compassion. Such quasi-Marxist theses of exploitation have been challenged by orthodox historians of psychiatry such as Kathleen Jones, but Foucault's term 'the great confinement' was certainly justified by the sheer weight of numbers of people deprived of their liberty in the asylum system. In England and Wales the total census of lunatic asylums showed an increase from four thousand inmates in the 1830s to seventy-four thousand by the end of the nineteenth century. This was quite disproportionate to the general increase in population over this period; the ratio of certified insane to overall population tripled from 9.18 per 10,000 of population in 1836, to 29.26 in 1890.[7]

Asylum doctors on lunar influence

The asylum was the domain of a new type of doctor: the alienist. Despite a paucity of medical treatments, leadership of the lunatic asylums was generally entrusted to physicians from the outset. Insanity obviously required

7   Figures from Scull (1979).

a quite different approach to the treatment of bodily disease, but the authorities, having been persuaded that lay management might expose lunatics to all kinds of abuse, saw in medical men informed judgement and moral integrity. In reality, asylum doctors were stifled by cheeseparing officialdom, their attention continually diverted to administering staff discipline and farm accounts. However, isolation of the insane in asylums provided opportunities for empirical study of behaviours and symptoms, enabling accrual of 'expertise and claims to expertise', and consequent professional autonomy. [8] Through observation, alienists such as Pinel and Johann Christian Reil (1759–1813) identified general patterns from the idiosyncrasies of individual cases. Their manuals laid the foundations of mental science — soon to be known as psychiatry.

This embryonic discipline dealt with an aspect of humanity thickly clothed in folklore. Although the term 'lunacy' was eschewed by alienists for its dubious derivation, so engrained was the lunar legend in society that the matter deserved investigation by asylum physicians. John Haslam, apothecary at the helm of the Bethlem Hospital in London from 1795 to 1816, had often heard reports of workhouse masters chaining and flogging inmates to prevent violence at full moon. In his *Observations on Madness and Melancholy*, Haslam stated that an exact register of cases under his observation over a two-year period showed no link between lunar cycles and mental excitement. While acknowledging that agitated persons were inevitably less likely to sleep when moonlight shone into their domiciles, he dismissed the notion as a figment of folklore, unworthy of further medical consideration.

However, increased excitement among inmates at new and full moon phases was observed by Michael Allen, superintendent at York Lunatic Asylum, and he produced intriguing data on temporal distribution of deaths. At this time, prior to effective treatment to quell acute mania, it was not uncommon for patients to die of exhaustion after a prolonged state of frenzy. As shown below, Allen's findings were not replicated in a larger survey by John Thurman at the nearby Retreat, based on 139 deaths over 44 years.

Table 4.1 Deaths in York mental establishments[9]

	Last quarter	New moon	First quarter	Full moon
Allen (York Lunatic Asylum)	3	15	1	11
Thurman (The Retreat)	32	40	34	33

Leading French alienists were receptive to *la croyance populaire*. The first observational study of asylum inmates was at the hospital for the insane in Chambery, by Joseph Daquin, whose positive findings led to his assertion in the respected textbook *Philosophie de la Folie* of 1791: 'it is a well established fact that insanity is a disease of the mind upon which the Moon exercises an unquestionable influence'.[10] Pinel believed that lunar cycles bore some influence on his patients, and Jean-Étienne Esquirol (1772–1840), his successor at the Salpêtrière mental hospital from 1810, urged an open mind in his widely read manual *Maladies Mentales*: 'An opinion which has existed for ages, which is spread abroad through all lands, and which is consecrated by finding a place in the vocabulary of every tongue, demands the most careful attention of observers.'[11]

Noting that Daquin had failed to use an objective measure of agitation, Leuret and Mitivié used the frequency of pulse as an indicator in their study at La Salpêtrière and Maison de Santé d'Ivry asylums (see below). They attributed differences between quarters to temperature changes.

Table 4.2 Pulse rates in mental patients at Salpêtrière and Maison de Santé d'Ivry[12]

	Last quarter	New moon	First quarter	Full moon
Pulse frequency	85.7	81.6	80.6	80.0
Patients with faster rate (%)	57.1	34.7	34.7	23.5

9 Figures from Laycock T (1843): 'On lunar influence; being a fourth contribution to proleptics'. *Lancet*, ii: 438-444.

10 Quoted by Esquirol (1837/1945). *Mental Maladies: Treatise on Insanity*. Translated from French, with additions, by EK Hunt. Philadelphia: Lea & Blanchard, p32.

11 Esquirol JD (1837/1845), p33.

12 Leuret F, Mitivié F (1832), *De la Fréquence du Pouls Chez les Aliénes*. Paris: Librairie Médicale de Crochard.

Esquirol stated that he had not been able to verify a lunar influence from his own observations, but remarked that the idea was taken seriously by Italian and German doctors. Across the Atlantic, Benjamin Rush (1746–1813), head of Pennsylvania State Hospital and venerated as the father of American psychiatry, examined the validity of the legend by ordering attendants to make detailed records of patients' behaviour. Finding few cases indicative of lunar timing, Rush explained that while atmospheric changes would have little effect on healthy people, rarefied air and increased light might excite individuals predisposed to episodes of mania, but whose numbers were too small to be noticed. Correspondingly, he believed some depressive types might worsen during periods of nocturnal darkness. A later study by SB Woodward of ninety cases at Worcester Asylum in Massachusetts produced little evidence of lunar association.

Erudite alienists may have followed developments in science and astronomy, and it was in the early nineteenth century that the Moon lost much of its remaining mystique. Telescopic scrutiny had satisfied most astronomers that the Moon was lifeless, despite popular imagination to the contrary. The authoritative text *Der Mond*, by German astronomers Wilhelm Beer (1797–1850) and Johann Mädler (1794–1874), described the Moon as devoid of water and air. However, early nineteenth century writers were aware of at least three direct actions of the Moon on Earth: as well as light and gravity, there was some degree of temperature modulation.

Traditionally people had believed that moonbeams had the opposite effect of the sun (a negative thermal association is indirectly true, in that the Moon shines brightest on clearer, cooler nights). Kepler had first stated that the Moon emits heat when lit by the sun, and analysis in the 1770s by Giuseppe Toaldo attributed an apparent meteorological influence of the Moon to reflection of sunrays. Early nineteenth-century astronomers concluded that the thermal effect is trivial, but traditional ideas prevailed, as in an astronomical calendar of 1809 by Hugh Rodger, describing various prognostic signs from the celestial bodies:

> If the moon look pale, look for rain; if fair and bright, fair weather; if red or blustring, storms or winds will ensue. The moon somewhat black or thick, provoketh rain; when the moon's horns is (sic) blunt at its rising, three days after the change, it denotes rainy weather for that quarter, but the other quarter seasonable weather.[13]

The weather certainly affected asylum admissions, with seasonal patterns in mania and melancholia, the former increasing in periods of warmth and light. Whereas the Sun was directly responsible through cases of insanity attributed to sunstroke, the meteorological influence of the Moon drew little interest from alienists. However, a lunar relationship with behaviour and illness was considered by distinguished English phy-

---

13   Rodger H (1809): *A Small Treatise of Astronomy*. Kilmarnock: H & S Crawford, p44.

sician Thomas Laycock. Best known for conceptualising the workings of the mind as physiological processes, Laycock wrote a series in *The Lancet* in the 1840s on proleptics (the prediction of human behaviour by environmental forces). Acknowledging the reports of Mead in the previous century as the beginnings of scholarly interest in lunar influence, Laycock described a 'vital periodity', a general law regulating all rhythms of animal life, observed in humans in menstruation, fevers, and paroxysmal disorders such as asthma and epilepsy, all of which appeared to coincide with lunar cycles.

Several alienists noted a link between menstruation and episodes of mania, and a weighty literature accumulated on uterine factors in female insanity, but despite its historical association with the menses, the Moon was rarely mentioned. However, a lunar pattern in migraine was suggested in an American medical dictionary of 1817, *hemicrania lunatica* denoting headaches caused by fluctuations in brain fluid according to phases of the Moon.[14] Swedish scientist Jöns Berzelius (1779–1848), famous for his work on chemical elements, and who named the metallic grey element selenium after the moon goddess, insisted that his attacks of migraine were timed by new and full moon. Visiting Paris in 1818 he was invited to dinner by the reputed mathematican-astronomer Laplace, who had laid a trap for him, ready with a French lunar calendar to refute the alleged causation. Berzelius had to decline the offer, spending the evening in bed in a dark room, unaware of the local phase of the Moon. Berzelius was mocked for his belief, but someone of his scientific standing could not be dismissed as an ignoramus.

The professional development of psychiatry

Asylum practice was a long way from the evidence-based doctrine of modern medicine. Drastic treatments were justified by early nineteenth-century alienists as a lesser evil to the ogre of insanity, but the efficacy of bleeding, surprise baths and spinning apparatus was theoretically dubious. American reformer Benjamin Rush made frequent use of the gyratory chair, believing that a swinging motion unblocked blood supply to the brain. Eventually, traumatising methods were curtailed, as the inspecting bodies expressed concern at abuses arguably worse than those originally

---

14   Coxe JR (1817): *The Philadelphia Medical Dictionary* (2nd edition). Philadelphia: Thomas Dobson & Son.

removed by lunacy reforms. Standardisation of asylum practice was based not on clinical evidence, but on a compromise of ethics and expedience.

Beyond the asylum walls, fads such as mesmerism and phrenology had failed to survive scrutiny, reinforcing the need for a mental science built on scientific rigour. Nineteenth century science was framed by positivism, a term coined by French philosopher Auguste Comte (1798–1857) for the Kantian synthesis of rationalism and empiricism. An anti-establishment thinker, Comte saw definitive knowledge as the means to solve the problems of society (and to overthrow regressive political systems); he instigated sociology as a scientific discipline. Alienists strove for acceptance as a credible branch of medicine, but in the rough terrain of mental science, the journey was tortuous. They were confronted by Cartesian dualism. Was the mind, unlike the corporeal brain, beyond empirical enquiry? The quest to understand mental disorder involved wider philosophical debate on the nature and spirit of human existence.

In attempting to reconcile natural and moral philosophy, John Stuart Mill, in his *System of Logic* of 1843, argued that although the mind was immaterial, its phenomena should be subjected to the same rules of enquiry as in the physical world. Alienists' literature shows how the pendulum of mind and brain in academic discourse swung towards a somatic construct. The professional journals launched in France, Germany and Britain in the mid-nineteenth century featured philosophical essays interspersed with anecdotal case reports, but pages were increasingly devoted to pathological enquiry. The ascendancy of positivism over metaphysical indulgences on the psyche was partly due to the constraints of asylum practice. Concentrated study of individual cases was precluded in hopelessly understaffed institutions, where the tenets of moral management seemed not only impractical, but therapeutically naïve. As a steady accumulation of chronic incurable cases demoralised doctors at the helm of asylums, a putative somatic root of insanity became the Holy Grail.

Meanwhile, a sense of alienation from the technocratic creed of industrial society had provoked an intellectual backlash. Progress, it seemed, was moving in a moral vacuum. The romantic movement was inspired by Jean Jacques Rousseau's *Noble Savage*, an epitome of innocent humanity untainted by the tyranny of organisation: 'man is born free, but everywhere he is in chains'.[15] In his resurrection of the soul, Rousseau had profound influence on the philosophy of Kant, Hegel, and Nietzsche; the creativity of Goethe, Delacroix and Beethoven; and on the triumphalism of Napoleon Bonaparte. Feelings were the expression of the true self, while reason was contrived—man had to rediscover himself. German philosophy was the bastion of a revival of the human spirit, and its psychiatry was undoubtedly influenced. In Kant's view, the study of human behaviour

---

15 Quoted in Almond B (1988): *Philosophy*. Harmondsworth: Penguin.

required an anthropological approach that could never become a rational or empirical science; Hegel (1770–1831) asserted that autonomy overrides instinct and imitation; for Friedrich Schelling (1775–1854), human unity with nature was the way to a higher plane of awareness, as expressed in the arts. Now Friedrich Nietzsche (1844–1900) was arguing that science denied man his own self and power.

German literature on insanity presented rich ontological debate between somaticists and psychicists, the latter inspired by late romanticism. In 1803 Johann Christian Reil wrote what is considered to be the first manual of psychotherapy: *Rhapsodien über die Anwendung der psychischen Curmethode auf Geisteszerrüttungen* (*Rhapsodies about the Application of Psychotherapy to Mental Disturbances*). Johann Christian Heinroth (1773–1843), from 1811 founding chair of the Institute for Psychological Medicine in Leipzig (the first school of psychiatry in the world), argued that mental illnesses were entirely afflictions of the soul. Influenced by the Protestant concepts of individual conscience and morality, Heinroth, in his *Lehrbuch der Störungen des Seelenlebens* (*Textbook on Disturbances of Mental Life*) of 1818, attributed insanity to inner conflict, leading to loss of free will. However, such works were not really precursors of psychoanalytic therapy, but a rationale for medical management and confinement in an asylum. Insanity was regarded as a loss of the very humanity of the individual, justifying drastic measures. Reil, who coined the term *psychiatrie* in 1808, emphasised fear as a therapeutic agent, and alienists continued to deploy shock methods. In mid-century, physician-philosophers Justinus Kerner and AKA von Eschenmeyer rekindled the fire of spiritual possession, recommending exorcism.

An instrumental figure in bridging the gap between philosophy and pathology was Wilhelm Griesinger (1817–1869). Having expertise in neurology, Griesinger sought to apprehend the inconveniently abstract phenomena of insanity. Accepting Hegel's argument that the higher faculties such as reasoning could not be located in physiology, Griesinger strove to synthesise mind and brain. He explained that mental disorder resulted not from physical or psychical cause alone, but from interaction between constitution and environment. Insanity was a disturbance to the equilibrium between a person and their surroundings, causing mental and neurological changes. Going against the grain, Griesinger unified insanity as a single disease (*Einheitpsychose*), with varying course and manifestations. His speculative concept of 'mentation', a behavioural product of underlying pathology, was criticised for its lack of empirical basis, but it paved the way for a fledgling profession from an incongruence of idealism and materialism towards a coherent body of knowledge.

In Britain the standard manual for many years was the *Treatise on Insanity* by James Cowles Prichard (1786–1848), a Bristol ethnologist and physician with a particular interest in nervous and mental disease. Prichard maintained the conventional categorisation of insanity by physical and moral causes, but even the latter were associated with pathological changes: social factors ultimately led to somatic damage. The succeeding core text was the *Manual of Psychological Medicine* of Bucknill and Tuke, first published in 1858, which placed greater emphasis on organic lesions; whether caused by bodily illness, lifestyle or environmental adversity, mental disorder developed as a neurological process. This was a time when epidemic illnesses such as cholera wreaked devastation, particularly in the urban lower class, and it was this segment of the populace that the lunatic asylums predominantly served. In their search for a microscopic causative agent of insanity, medical superintendents introduced laboratories, and post-mortem investigations became routine. As well as examining the hemispheres of the brain, alienists dissected visceral organs, the digestive tract being particularly suspected. Such endeavours, largely fruitless, waned after the great watershed of 1859, when Charles Darwin unleashed the theory of evolution.

Tainted stock

The idea of organic evolution could be traced back to ancient Greece. Ionian scholar Anaximander, on noting mammalian properties in a shark, had reckoned that all living creatures began as fish, before evaporation by the Sun created dry land. However, the process lacked a credible mechanism. For some decades, Jean-Baptiste Lamarck (1744–1829) had provided the prevailing wisdom on hereditary passage. In Lamarckian theory, attributes were acquired: giraffes gained their long necks from stretching, injury to a creature's limb would be reflected in its offspring. Returning from his Latin American voyages on the *Beagle*, Charles Darwin (1809–1882) formulated his theory of natural selection, but he was tardy in publishing, and only the threat of losing priority to a competing naturalist spurred him into action. Following his studies in the Amazon basin and Malay archipelago, by the mid-1850s Alfred Russel Wallace (1823–1913) was describing the evolutionary process as a tree continually branching out, dividing into new twigs. According to Wallace, survival of species was determined not by chance, but by suitability for the environment. Under pressure, Darwin's theory of evolution was hastily released, under the full title *On the Origin of Species by Means of Natural Selection, or the Preservation of Favoured Races in the Struggle for Life.*

The book had sensational impact. Here was the law explaining the form of every organism, from the camouflage of a beetle to the human brain; by attributing a common ancestry to every beast, Darwin demolished anthropocentric assumptions. As diversification of species required millions of years, the theory of evolution indicated that both *terra* and *homo sapiens* were very much older than the Scriptures taught. Scientific estimates of the age of the Earth had increased dramatically in the previous century, when Comte de Buffon suggested that the Earth was a moulted rock resulting from a comet striking the Sun. Buffon calculated how long the Earth would have taken to cool enough to support life. His figure of 75,000 years was soon surpassed by fellow Frenchman Jean Fourier, who took account of the insulating effect on cooling of the solid core, but the latter's estimate of 100 million years was still well short of the currently accepted duration of 4,500 million years.

Emboldened propagandists of scientific materialism were confidently witnessing the 'long withdrawing roar' of the tide of Christianity, as mourned in Matthew Arnold's (1867) poem *Dover Beach*. The floodgates opened on waters already swollen by radical philosophers. Bavarian critical theologian Ludwig Feuerbach (1804–1872) had urged the liberation of human consciousness from religious fantasy, while Karl Marx had described faith as 'the opium of the masses'. Later in the century, Sigmund Freud (1856–1939) would dismiss faith as an infantilism on mankind's path to maturity. Amidst high Darwinism, evangelical Henry Drummond coined the phrase 'God of the Gaps' for the erroneous notion that as scientific horizons expanded, the realm of divinity would diminish.[16] Yet Darwin himself was no standard bearer, leaving others to teleological debate. His position was agnostic, a term introduced by TH Huxley, the 'attack dog' of Darwin's theory. Evolution had not explained creation, only the subsequent pattern of progression. However, no scientific theory had so drastically undermined faith; just as cosmology had precluded divine control of the stars, now sublunary anarchy was brought under universal law.

Evolutionary principles gave impetus to anthropology, the study of biological and cultural development, which had its heyday in the late nineteenth century. Many an expedition was made to remote equatorial forests and Pacific islands, to the habitat of primitive societies untouched by modern civilisation. Among the diverse peoples subjected to the gaze of bearded investigators, animistic myth and moon lore were prominent. Comte in his *Cours de Philosophie Positive* of 1830 had presented a grand narrative of three stages of human development. In the theological phase phenomena were attributed to supernatural powers; the metaphysical stage was concerned with mysterious atmospheric forces; and finally

16   Drummond H (1904): *The Lowell Lectures on the Ascent of Man*. Glasgow: Hodder & Stoughton.

mankind had entered the scientific stage, with knowledge based on empirically validated theory. According to Comte, the attribution of spiritual powers to inanimate objects was a pre-religious stage, indicating an enormous rift in human development between the primitive and industrialised world. *Die Theologie ist die Anthropologie*, argued Feuerbach.

A linear process was also described by Oxford anthropologist Edward B Tylor (1832–1917), whose work *Primitive Culture* of 1871 fitted mythology into a Darwinian progression in human thought. In his monogenist model, all human races had common origin, but were at different stages on the same path. Tylor's observations influenced 'armchair anthropologist' JG Frazer, author of several volumes under the title *The Golden Bough*, who charted human development from magic through religion to science. However, the assumed retarded status of aboriginal society was rejected by philosopher Herbert Spencer (1820–1903), who explained that rituals were based on rational belief systems forged from the duality of natural and supernatural. Inextricable from context, myth was thus an element of reality in a specific social system.

Indeed, supernatural ideas persisted in western society, illustrating the cultural lag between scientific advances and their diffusion into lay knowledge. Although the wrath of the stars was no longer feared, Reverend Timothy Harley in his compendium *Moon Lore* noted the widespread persistence of lunar mythology: 'In the nineteenth century as well as in the dark ages, in London as well as in the ends of the earth, men of all colours and clans are found turning their faces heavenward to read their duty and destiny in the oracular face of the moon.'[17]

Harley described a plethora of surviving lunar legends in rural counties. For example, there was a saying in Huntingdonshire that 'a dark Christmas sends a fine harvest';[18] while country dwellers in France and Germany believed that sleeping in moonlight was hazardous. Perceived powers of the moon were strongest among farmers and fishermen, whose livelihoods were most directly affected by the forces of nature. That such conviction was not restricted to the scientifically naïve drew scorn from Edward Tylor:

> The notion that the weather changes with the moon's quarterings is still held with great vigour in England. That educated people to whom exact weather records are accessible should still find satisfaction in the fanciful lunar rule, is an interesting case of intellectual survival.[19]

In popular culture, belief in the Moon as harbinger of madness remained strong. Many a relative would insist that the mental derange-

17   Harley T (1885): *Moon Lore*. London: Swan Sonnenschein, Le Bas & Lowry, p176.
18   Harley (1885), p181.
19   Tyler EB (1873): *Primitive Culture*. London: Watts.

ment of a newly admitted patient fluctuated with lunar cycles, as noted by one nineteenth-century asylum superintendent in England:

> Among the uneducated, the most remarkable opinion which still con-
> tinues to maintain its ground is that of the moon's influence on insan-
> ity. When patients are conveyed to the hospitals, their friends,
> especially if they come from the country, generally state them to be
> worse at some particular period of the moon.[20]

Applied to the social development of mankind, the theory of evolution had major impact on psychiatry. Predating Darwin's 1871 text *The Descent of Man* was the independently devised thesis of Herbert Spencer, whose *Principles of Psychology* of 1855 had introduced the phrase 'survival of the fittest'. Spencer espoused *laissez-faire* principles, believing that while state welfare counteracted the natural struggle for existence, evolution would ultimately favour the intelligent. However, pessimism was rife in Victorian society, as the inexorable growth of the uneducated masses threatened to overturn social order and reverse the progress of civilisation. In the early days of the Industrial Revolution, Thomas Malthus (1766–1834) had warned that whereas population grew at a geometric ratio, food production could only rise on an arithmetical scale. The privileged stratum feared being overwhelmed. Meanwhile, some anthropologists considered human development as a racial hierarchy, according to how primitive or ape-like members of tribes or races appeared. John Langdon-Down (1828–1896), renowned for identifying the eponymous syndrome, in which he assimilated the appearance of those afflicted to a Mongolian, had 'no doubt that these ethnic features are the result of degeneration'.[21] The lowest level of mental defective, known as 'idiots' (in current terminology, people with severe learning difficulty), were seen by some asylum physicians as half-way between animal and human.

Admissions to asylums suggested mental defect running in families, and hereditary determinism became a prominent theme in the aetiology of insanity, as in the prolific writings of British psychiatrist Henry Maudsley (1835–1918). Physical and mental degeneracy were increasingly blamed on an inheritance of vice including alcohol abuse, immorality and illegitimate offspring. With the inferred intractability of insanity, the role of the asylum changed from unrealistic curative endeavour to preventing procreation of tainted stock. This was a cause conveniently served by the institutional regime, with its strict gender segregation. Evolutionary theory was later fused with genetics, a science emerging from the rediscovery of the work of monk Gregor Mendel (1822–1884). Meticulous experiments by

20   Anonymous (1850): *Familiar Views of Lunacy and Lunatic Life: With Hints on the Personal Care and Management of Those who are Afflicted with Temporary or Permanent Derangement*. London: John W Parker.
21   Quoted in Ryan J, Thomas F (1980): *The Politics of Mental Handicap*. Harmondsworth: Penguin, p105.

Mendel in the abbey garden of Brünn had revealed distinct, binary factors in peas, which were dominant or recessive in transmission. His findings, published in 1866, drew little interest at the time, but further research conducted decades after his death confirmed a mechanism unknown to Darwin. Genes were discovered as the submicroscopic units of heredity, producing evolutionary change through random mutations. As moral and environmental factors became secondary to the immutable laws of genetics, many psychiatrists became enthusiasts of eugenics, a term coined by Victorian polymath Francis Galton, a cousin of Charles Darwin, for racial improvement by judicious mating. The potential of human engineering was notoriously applied in the sterilisation programme for the mentally subnormal in California, and the mass extermination of mental defectives in Nazi Germany.

Mania and the Moon

The concept of lunacy was conspicuous by its absence from psychiatric literature, until a lengthy report on the influence of the Moon by German psychiatrist Friedrich Koster, spread over three editions of the *Allgemeine Zeitschrift für Psychiatrie* in 1859 and 1860. Such a prestigious journal may have risked its reputation by affording so much space to a discredited idea, but this article was clearly the product of careful observational research. Koster had amassed over six years of data at Marsberg, a former monastery converted in 1814 to the Provinzial-Irrenenstalt Westfälen (Provincial Mental Asylum for Westphalia). Moreover, Koster's work, published as *Untersuchungen über den Einfluss des Mondes auf das periodische Irresein* (*On the Influence of the Moon on Periodic Insanity*) related to a topical issue of the time: the relationship between mania and depression.

Psychiatrists were beginning to delineate the occurrence of episodes of mania and melancholia in the same patient as a distinct, often cyclical illness. Early in the asylum era Pinel had observed that insanity was most commonly episodic in presentation, and in his *Maladies Mentales* Esquirol described *folie continue, remittent* and *intermittente*. In 1845 Griesinger referred to alternating mania and depression as *cyclus* in his textbook *Mental Pathology and Therapeutics*. In the 1850s, when Koster was beginning his research, French alienists Jean-Pierre Falret and Jules Baillarger offered slightly differing conceptualisations of a cyclical condition, named *folie circulaire* and *folie à double forme* respectively.[22] While the taxonomic debate ensued, Koster hypothesised a relationship of intermittent mania to lunar cycles. Drawing on the earlier observations of Mead, Koster anticipated correlation between manic episodes and the proximity of the Moon. Among the detailed case studies was Frau Thun, a 48-year-old mother of three, admitted in 1855 after bouts of mania and melancholia. Her spells of mania regularly occurred at approach of apogee, while her depressed episodes lasted from apogee to perigee. Koster did not conclude direct causation, but suggested that body rhythms coincide with lunar cycles. Koster, who became director of the asylum in 1860, continued his longitudinal research, his findings collated in a book *Die Gesetze des periodischen Irreseins*, published in 1882. Judging by a lack of coverage in journal reviews, Koster's work had little impact within his profession.

Eminent alienist Forbes Benignus Winslow (1810–1874), who in 1848 had launched the *Journal of Psychological Medicine* (the first British psychiatric journal), remarked on lunar influence in 1867 in his monograph *Light: its Influence on Life and Health*. While regarding the hypothesis as highly speculative, and acknowledging that the claims of Pinel, Daquin and Guislain were no longer supported by practitioners, Winslow was not inclined to issue any firm conclusions on an unsatisfactorily investigated phenomenon. Intrigued by the insistence of the matron of his private asylum that patients were more agitated at full moon, Winslow suggested that apparent lunar patterns in mental conditions of periodicity may be due to meteorological conditions on Earth moderated by the Moon, including rarity of air, electrical atmosphere, heat, moisture and wind. He was inclined to regard changes in nocturnal brightness as the main factor.

By the end of the century, only sporadic references to the Moon appeared in psychiatric literature. Daniel Hack Tuke in his celebrated *Dictionary of Psychological Medicine* included an entry on the lunar legend, stating that no positive evidence had emerged since Esquirol's time. Italian psychiatrist and criminologist Cesare Lombroso (1836–1909), controversial for his theory of a biologically distinct criminal type identifiable by physiognomy, ardently believed in a lunar effect on behaviour. One of the last psychiatric textbooks to afford any serious mention of the Moon was a clinical manual of 1907 by George Savage, ex-superintendent of the Bethlem Hospital, who noted that while asylum attendants talked of a mystical lunar effect, the link would be entirely explained by illumination. 'Has the moon really anything to do with insanity? My opinion is, that

---

22 Bipolar affective disorder, as the condition is now known, is discussed at greater length in Chapter 8.

many lunatics will remain quiet in bed during darkness, but will be mischievous and refractory if there is light enough.'[23]

Epilepsy and the ether

Marked by their protective leather skull caps, large numbers of people with epilepsy were confined alongside the insane. This was not only for administrative convenience, but justified by the extremely troublesome behaviour of such patients, for whom an explosion of maniacal violence was the most common route to the asylum. The first major studies of the disease took place in Parisian lunatic asylums, where Esquirol defined *grand mal* and *petit mal* seizures. In his manual on insanity, Esquirol presented findings from the case histories of 385 women from an epileptic ward. After omitting forty-six found to have feigned epilepsy or hysteria, all but a fifth of his heterogenous sample had mental disorder of some form. The condition *furor epilepticus* was of particular interest to Esquirol, a crazed state sometimes lasting several days, in which patients often attacked others savagely and indiscriminately. The extent of behavioural overlap led alienists to interpret epilepsy and insanity as basically the same condition, with Thomas Clouston suggesting a common pathology. Griesinger observed that mania in epileptic patients tended to progress to irreversible insanity (then known as 'dementia'). Over several decades alienists toyed with the direction of relationship: did epilepsy cause insanity, or vice versa?

Deciphering the mechanism of epilepsy was impossible before the demystification of electricity and its role in human physiology. In the previous century, great advances had been made in understanding this invisible force. Benjamin Franklin's experiments had differentiated positive and negative electricity, and Charles Coulomb had demonstrated that the interaction between two charges followed a similar rule to Newton's law of gravity. In 1791 came a revelation from Bologna, where anatomist Luigi Galvani claimed to have discovered 'animal electricity' in laboratory experiments on frogs, although this was refuted two years later by Alessandro Volta, who showed how the muscle contractions had resulted from contact with different metals. Animal electricity was dismissed as a restatement of vitalism. Nonetheless, the accidental connections between Galvani's electrical apparatus and scalpel had revealed a new form of electricity– the steady current. Forty years passed before the existence of

---

23   Savage GH, Goodall E (1907): *Insanity and Allied Neuroses: A Practical and Clinical Manual.* London: Cassell.

bioelectrical activity was confirmed using the galvanometer, with impulses detected in nerve cells. This was the time of the amateur scientific enterprise of bookbinder's apprentice Michael Faraday (1791–1867), who revealed the inextricable link between electricity and magnetism. Faraday's concept of the force field was the catalyst for the electromagnetic wave theory of James Clerk Maxwell, whose equations in turn led to Einstein's theory of relativity.

Bioelectricity became an exciting new field of medical research, and the workings of the brain came to be understood as an ongoing sequence of electrical sparks.[24] Acquainted with Faraday was Robert Bentley Todd (1809–1860), a physician at King's College Hospital in London. Todd postulated electromagnetic polarity in the nervous system, and his experiments on rabbits showed that seizures arose from abnormal electrical discharge in the brain. He presented his findings to the Royal College of Physicians in 1849, but the work was not widely disseminated, and it was John Hughlings Jackson (1835–1911) who took much of the credit for illuminating the physiological process of epilepsy. Jackson had worked under Thomas Laycock in York before making his name at the National Hospital for the Paralysed and Epileptic at Queen's Square, London. This was the first neurological hospital in the world, its opening in 1860 spurred by the presence of epilepsy in the Royal Family. Best known for his work on function and localisation in epilepsy, Jackson was instrumental in establishing epilepsy as an organic syndrome. He explained a seizure as 'an occasional, sudden, massive, rapid and local discharge of the grey matter',[25] although he initially failed to acknowledge the electrical basis of this explosive activity. For some years Jackson worked at the laboratory of the West Riding Pauper Lunatic Asylum, where he described various paroxysmal events observed in inmates as miniature seizures.

As no lesion in the cerebral cortex could be located, idiopathic epilepsy remained loosely defined. With manifestations encompassing not only convulsions but also behavioural changes, epilepsy continued to be regarded as a neurosis by many nineteenth-century neurologists; they believed that extreme emotional stimulation had a generalised impact on the nervous system, causing seizures. Epilepsy was conflated with hysteria, both conditions showing tendencies for excessive sensitivity, religious absolutism and irrational hostility. Indeed, the first pharmacological anticonvulsant, announced in 1857 by English neurologist Charles Locock, arose from experimental use of bromides in women with hysteria. Hughlings Jackson observed a range of postictal[26] mental states from mild

---

24 Message relay in the nervous system was eventually revealed as an electrochemical process in the 1920s.

25 Quoted in Scott D (1969) *About Epilepsy*. London: Duckworth, p98.

26 The suffix '-ictal' means seizures; 'postictal' is the immediate aftermath.

confusion to maniacal frenzy, but in his psycho-physical parallelism, all psychological features of epilepsy were manifestations of physical processes, and he dismissed the psychogenic condition of hystero-epilepsy. Distinguished Parisian neurologist Jean Martin Charcot (1825–1893), who spent most of his career at La Salpêtrière asylum, learned much from observing hysteria and epilepsy in the wards, finding that the fits of the former were merely an imitation of the paroxysmal attacks of the latter. Charcot thus made an important distinction between organic epilepsy and its psychogenic relation.

Neurologists had shown that mental deterioration was not a normal complication of epilepsy, and that only a small proportion of sufferers exhibited significant psychological disturbance. Mental disorder, therefore, was not pathognomonic; the epileptic inmates of asylums were not representative of the general syndrome. However, epilepsy remained a significant concern for alienists. The condition of epileptic insanity was established in 1860 by Jules Falret, who categorised mental disturbance as peri-ictal, interictal and chronic. He shared his interest in epilepsy with Benedict Morel, director of a nearby asylum, and they often visited patients together. Morel regarded irritability and angry outbursts as fundamental features of an epileptic personality. As well as cases of troublesome and aggressive behaviour either before or after convulsions, Falret identified a psychic form of epileptic insanity whereby seizures were substituted by recurring delirious states, often with concomitant violence. In his book *Body and Mind*, leading British psychiatrist Henry Maudsley accepted Morel's concept, describing how in some cases maniacal outbursts recurred regularly for several years before true seizures presented: 'Instead of the morbid action affecting the motor centres and issuing in a paroxysm of convulsions, it fixes upon the mind-centres and issues in a paroxysm of mania, which is, so to speak, an epilepsy of mind.'[27]

For asylum attendants, the epileptic insane were particularly awkward to manage, requiring observation day and night for seizures, and having propensity to violence. Maudsley regarded them as the most dangerous cases, marked by psychopathic impulses and a destructive frenzy following seizures. Unpredictability was exemplified by the epileptic artist Vincent van Gogh, who had several admissions to an asylum: during one attack he cut off one of his ears. Patients were assigned to wards on the basis of conduct, and epileptics were often accommodated in the dormitories for the noisy and truculent. GF Barham, writing in 1907, portrayed Ward K, the epileptic ward at Claybury Hospital near London, as a volatile environment. Fights were as frequent as fits, with the potentially fatal *status epilepticus* a regular event. Seclusion in padded rooms was frequently required. Yet epileptic patients were also useful to the asylum.

27   Maudsley H (1873) *Body and Mind*. London: Macmillan, p247.

Having long spells of lucidity between attacks, their labour was a boon to the farm and workshops of the institution, and physical exertion was believed to reduce the frequency of seizures. The average proportion of epileptics in asylums remained around 10 per cent by the early twentieth century, but in recognition of their special needs, separate institutions began to appear, particularly in the USA. In Britain, Ewell Epileptic Colony in Surrey opened in 1900, where a productive farm served neighbouring London County Council asylums.

While the possibility of lunar influence was scarcely mentioned in the burgeoning literature on epilepsy, prominent late nineteenth-century neurologist William Gowers attributed temporal seizure patterns to menstrual cycles. Environmental stimuli were also considered. Thanks to Faraday and the physicist James Clerk Maxwell (1831–1879), originator of the theory of electromagnetism, the clockwork universe described by the scientific materialists of the Enlightenment had been displaced by a complexity of waves and force fields. The effects of extraterrestrial forces on behaviour were studied by Swedish scientist Svante Arrhenius (1859–1927), who was later awarded the Nobel Prize in Chemistry (and honoured by a lunar crater). In his paper *Cosmic Influences on Physiological Phenomena* in 1898, analysis of nine thousand epileptic seizures showed correlation with lunar phases, as did births, deaths and menses. Arrhenius attributed the higher frequency of epileptic fits at bedtime and waking to atmospheric changes at these times of day, a conclusion in accord with neurologist Georg Lomer's finding from detailed study of seven cases that the epileptic brain lacked flexibility to barometric fluctuation. According to Arrhenius, air pressure was indirectly regulated by the Moon through its rhythmic influence on the electrical field.

Epileptic inmates being particularly sensitive to environmental stress, Ernest White, superintendent of the City of London Asylum at Dartford, studied various excitatory factors, including lunar phases. Over a two-year period to 1900, he found that fits peaked just after full moon, but only in females. Evidently this was unrelated to menstruation. White remarked on the general belief in asylums that chronic inmates were more agitated and destructive at full moon, citing a steward at his institution whose proof was in the amount of broken crockery. Yet the copious records of seizures gathered at asylums and neurology clinics did not suggest temporal patterns of clinical import, and conjecture on the impact of atmospheric or ethereal forces, whether or not related to the Moon, occupied few columns of the literature on epilepsy.

An observational deficit

Since the mid-nineteenth century, Germany had built a reputation as the international seat of psychiatry, a mantle held until the Third Reich. Of all the genius nurtured by its prestigious university clinics, the most enduring name is that of Emil Kraepelin (1856–1926), founder of modern psychiatric classsification. Until the 1890s, the nosology of psychiatry was a conceptual fog of imprecisely defined syndromes, tautologies and obfuscation of causes and symptoms. Kraepelin, whose rigid mindset inclined towards Teutonic supremacism, devoted his career to placing his discipline on a proper scientific footing. Wary of interpretative formulations, his mission was to build the subject matter of psychiatry into a descriptive, hierarchical structure. He devised a coherent classification of insanity, delineating natural diseases of distinct courses and symptomatic profiles, gradually refined over many editions of his textbook *Psychiatrie*. The severest form, psychosis, he divided into dementia praecox manic-depressive and epileptic types. Kraepelin advised psychiatrists not to waste time in understanding how patients felt, but to concentrate on accurate diagnosis. His taxonomy fulfilled a yearning for order among peers, but many psychiatrists thought his prognostic certainties dogmatic and sterile.

Dementia praecox was renamed 'schizophrenia' by his contemporary Eugen Bleuler, who saw the condition not as a life sentence but as an affliction of the psyche amenable to therapeutic intervention. Swiss émigré Adolph Meyer (1866–1950), who emerged as leader of American psychiatry in the interwar years, eschewed Kraepelin's depersonalising schema. Instead, Meyer emphasised the unique biography of the patient, and at Johns Hopkins University he transformed psychiatric training with his psychobiology model, which conceptualised mental disorders as 'reaction types'. However, while individualism was feasible in the United States, where the majority of psychiatrists were in private practice, it was impractical in the state mental hospital. Kraepelin had provided a credible diagnostic framework, but for psychiatry to tag closer to the flotilla of the medical model, it needed effective treatment.

The first oasis in a therapeutic desert was in 1918, when Julius Wagner von Jauregg (1857–1940) discovered a malarial remedy for general paralysis of the insane, a neurosyphilitic condition that was a leading cause of death in asylums. This heralded a physical onslaught on the great dragons of psychiatry, schizophrenia and manic-depressive psychosis. Psychiatrists envisaged a brave new world of active treatment and discharge, and in the 1930s a multitude of patients were exposed indiscriminately to the ravages of insulin coma therapy, chemically-induced seizures and psychosurgery. However, the so-called shock treatments transpired as a false dawn, and the population of mental institutions continued to rise. Despite gradual increases in medical staffing, doctors faced an insurmountable task. Recently admitted patients might see a psychiatrist every week, but the legions of chronic cases were left to the back wards, where an overworked nursing staff maintained a stultifying regime.

Having ongoing contact with patients day and night, it was mostly the nurses who observed and managed behaviour. Until the 1960s, mental nursing was an arduous vocation of long hours, strict discipline and poor pay; the majority of nurses lived on the asylum estate with restricted leave. Such work attracted a barely educated class, typically from rural backwaters and Ireland, where work opportunities were few. In the isolated asylum culture, nurses were carriers of folklore from the dales and *glenns*, and the legendary powers of the Moon were inevitably embellished and projected on to their charges. With nurses lacking inclination or capacity for systematic investigation, accounts of a lunar impact on patients remained entirely anecdotal. As Chung and Nolan explained in their historical review of mental health nursing, while nurses observed, only the intellectually superior doctors could interpret.[28] As first-hand witnesses, nurses were grossly neglected in the literature on mental hospital care, and observations of lunar influence would have been confined to ward banter. The beginnings of proper investigation into the influence of the Moon on mental patients would rely on investigators from beyond the walls of the asylum.

In the late nineteenth century, a new discipline emerged. While having rather disparate structure in its formative decades, psychology began to divide into two sharply contrasting paradigms, with one side defining itself as the study of behaviour and the other as the study of mind. The latter was the psychoanalytic movement instigated by Freud, which delved into unconscious drives, typically attributing symptoms to unresolved childhood conflict. The impetus of Freud and his followers gained momentum after the Great War, when the positivist hereditary-organic model of psychiatry was challenged by the legions of previously healthy young men suffering from 'shell-shock', a hysterical rather than concussive condition resulting from prolonged exposure to the terrors of trench warfare. Psychotherapeutic intervention was famously applied by WHR Rivers at Craiglockhart in Edinburgh to traumatised officers including war poets Siegfried Sassoon and Wilfred Owen. The traditional stigma towards mental disorder softened in the wave of sympathy for the shat-

---

28   Chung MC, Nolan P (1994): 'The influence of positivistic thought on nineteenth century nursing'. *Journal of Advanced Nursing*, 19: 226-232.

tered souls returning from the Western Front: they deserved treatment, not incarceration.

The psychoanalytic movement, however, made little inroads to the therapeutically impoverished asylums (now renamed 'mental hospitals'), where the majority of long-term residents did not have treatable neuroses but schizophrenia, involutional melancholia, senile dementia and general paralysis of the insane. With the notable exception of the psychodynamic work of Harry Stack Sullivan at Chestnut Lodge, few psychiatrists of analytic bent ventured into the psychotic wilderness. A combination of resource constraints and ideological hostility kept the 'cult' of Freud and Jung outside the walls of institutional psychiatry. Nonetheless, psychoanalytic theory had widespread impact on intellectual discourse of the early to mid-twentieth century, providing insights to the apparent crisis of civilisation and the inherent destructiveness of individual and society.

In its formulations of mind and motive, psychoanalytic literature offered new perspectives on the relationship between human being and cosmos. Repressed infantile sexuality was the dominant theme of Freudian analysis, and the Moon was understood as a potent libido symbol, as discussed by WA White in the journal *Psychoanalytic Review* in 1914. The mythological male sun/female moon dichotomy was revived in the analytic psychology of Carl Gustav Jung. Accused of occultism by Freud, Jung regarded spirituality as a necessary opposite to reason, within a collective as well as individual unconscious. In dreams, which Jung regarded as a means of adjustment to the psychological conflict of everyday life, the Moon in its phases presented a primordial analogy of life, death and rebirth. Isidor Sadger in 1920 described 'moonstruck' sleepwalkers who rose from bed, sometimes being lured outdoors, to stare at the luminous sphere. This form of somnambulism had appeared earlier in the annals of psychiatry, Ebers in 1838 having described a case of an 11-year-old boy in Breslau whose wanderings coincided with full moon, and in Germany the term *Mondsucht* was a byword for madness. Sadger explained that the Moon aroused sexual memories of the mother's breast. Hungarian psychotherapist Francis Völgyesi in his *Message to the Neurotic World* noted that on certain days patients with epilepsy or of nervous disposition converged on his consulting room in states of irritability and low mood, finding that 'upon such an accumulation of complaints I glance at the calendar and find that there is a new moon'.[29]

Despite its use of scientific terminology, psychoanalytic theory lacked validation of its speculative and often obscurantist propositions, and its encroachment on mainstream psychiatry provoked antipathy. The physical treatments of the 1930s boosted the biological model and laid the foun-

---

29   Völgyesi F (1935): *A Message to the Neurotic World*. Translated from Hungarian by B Balogh. London: Hutchinson & Co., p74.

dations for evidence-based practice, to which psychoanalysts could not contribute. Psychiatrists, however, were rather more receptive to the other arm of psychology, which had robust empirical credentials. Experimental psychology was born in the 1880s, when pioneers swept aside the last vestiges of romanticism to develop a science of human behaviour. Wilhelm Wundt (1832–1920) wrote *Principles of Physiological Psychology*, regarded as the first textbook of psychology, and established the first psychological laboratory in Leipzig. William James (1842–1910), a protagonist of the philosophy of pragmatism, was a major figure in the development of the nascent discipline. Psychology, he bemoaned, was barely beyond the stage of physics before Galileo, and of chemistry before Lavoisier. Rejecting the subject-object dualism that had constrained investigation into abstract, higher mental faculties, James regarded the mind as an expression of ongoing adjustment to the physical and social environment. All psychical activity was a manifestation of neurophysiology, with feelings mere 'epiphenomena'. In 1892 he reflected: 'I wished, by treating Psychology *like* a natural science, to help her to become one.'[30]

Regarding 'mind', 'meaning', and 'will' as quaint ideas from a pre-scientific outlook, experimental psychologists focused entirely on observable behaviour, on which propositions could be tested by scientific method. Emotions were not conducive to deterministic law, but probabilistic statements could be generated on relationships between behavioural variables, and this led to the development of standardised rating scales and statistical techniques. Whereas nineteenth century philosophers had regarded the immaterial mind as beyond scientific investigation, empiricist psychology promised to reduce all mental processes to objectively measurable categories. Their intellectual champion was Francis Galton (1822–1911), who declared that 'until the phenomena of any branch of knowledge have been submitted to measurement and number, it cannot assume the dignity of a science'.[31] Galton's work was continued by the founder of modern statistics, Karl Pearson (1857–1936). Best known today for his eponymous tests of correlation, Pearson saw statistics as the fundamental basis of every branch of science. In his *Grammar of Science*, initially appearing in 1892, he stated that 'the material of science is coextensive with the whole life, physical and mental, of the universe'.[32] Following his animal learning experiments in Massachusetts, Edward Lee Thorndike (1874–1949) argued that if social and psychological phenomena exist, they must exist to a numerical degree and therefore be amenable to quantitative analysis. His *Introduction to the Theory of Mental and Social Measurements*,

30   James W (1892): 'A plea for psychology as a "natural science"'. *Philosophical Reviews*, 1: 146–153.
31   Galton F (1879): 'Psychometric experiments'. *Brain*, 2: 149–162.
32   Pearson K (1911) *The Grammar of Science* (3rd edition) London: A & C Black.

first published in 1904, was the prescriptive text for the fledgling social and behavioural sciences.

Thus psychology, unlike the clinical pragmatism of psychiatry, pursued its professional project through rigorous scientific methodology. Initially operating at the margins of the mental hospital system, clinical psychologists were gradually afforded a role in assessment, administering their standardised instruments to measure cognition, perception, personality traits, intelligence and learning.[33] By assisting the psychiatrist with assessment and elements of the treatment plan, and with their skills in research, psychologists got their foot in the door, and went on to pursue their professional project of achieving equal status with medical practitioners (in which they have achieved limited success). With their statistical prowess and methodical zeal, could psychologists determine whether lunacy is fact or fantasy?

---

33 Psychologist and historian John Hall, in a lecture entitled 'New Kids on the Block' at the Institute of Psychiatry, King's College London (9 November 2010) emphasised that clinical psychology in Britain had no single model or professional organisation until later in the twentieth century. With typical vanity Hans Eysenck at the Maudsley Hospital claimed that he single-handedly developed clinical psychology as a discipline, but its expansion was very slow. In 1970 Hall was appointed as a research assistant at the huge mental institution at Wakefield, Yorkshire, where input was restricted to two sessions per week by a clinical psychologist from the nearby prison (and that was for a research project).

Five

An elusive proof

The high water mark of the asylum population was reached in the mid-1950s. Thereafter, in Britain, USA and throughout the developed world, the human tide began to recede. The impetus of deinstitutionalisation has often been attributed to the 'wonder drugs' for schizophrenia, but chlorpromazine (branded Largactil) arrived when the resident population was already falling. It had long been appreciated that the dreaded asylum was not the ideal environment for recovery from mental breakdown. Separate units had been built in the grounds of British mental hospitals since the 1930s, following legislation permitting voluntary admission for new, treatable cases. Only patients with intractable conditions would then have the misfortune to graduate to the institution proper.

After the Second World War, inspired by the work of psychiatrist Maxwell Jones with refugees, the therapeutic community model was introduced, with its four tenets of communality, permissiveness, democracy and reality confrontation. While the old custodial order was softening in hospitals with progressive medical leadership, change was a slow process. The rigid institutional culture was exposed by several ethnographic studies, particularly in the USA, showing how the individual needs of patients were overriden by administrative convenience.[1] Sociologist Erving Goffman spent months at a mammoth New York state mental hospital, observing a tendency for nurses of this 'total institution' to preserve existential distance from patients, as a defence against stigma. British psychiatrist Russell Barton described 'institutional neurosis', an iatrogenic condition superimposed on the patient's underlying disorder by the depersonalising, ritualistic *milieu*. Clearly the mental hospital was in need of overhaul, and the breakthrough of tranquillisers boosted the momentum. Doors were unlocked in the darkest corners of the asylum, leaving a few secure wards on male and female sides, airing court fences were dis-

---

1   One of the most insightful was by Stanton AH and Schwartz MS (1954): *The Mental Hospital*. New York: Basic Books.

mantled, trusted patients were given more liberal parole, and modern industrial workshops brought a semblance of normality to hospital life.

The Largactil revolution, unlike the uncritically accepted physical treatments of the 1930s, was based on high standards of scientific appraisal. Until the mid-twentieth century evaluation was rather cursory throughout medicine, with treatments often introduced on what would today be considered dubious evidence. A notorious example in psychiatry was prefrontal leucotomy, the surgical severing of cerebral fibres that thwarted troublesome behaviour but permanently blunted the patient's personality. Hundreds of thousands of patients across the world were subjected to this destructive and sometimes fatal operation based on cavalier reports of startling improvements. In the 1950s more sophisticated methodology, combined with higher ethical standards, transformed medical research.

The experimental method was born at sea in the eighteenth century, when countless sailors died of scurvy, a wasting disease for which there was no known remedy. James Lind, surgeon on HMS *Salisbury*, isolated twelve sufferers and divided them into pairs for six possibly antiscorbutic treatments: cyder, elixir of vitriol, vinegar, sea water, nutmeg paste, and citrus fruit. The men stayed in the same compartment, with an otherwise uniform diet. Those taking oranges and lemons rapidly recovered and returned to duty, whereas the others showed temporary improvement at most. The results were indisputable, and once the British Admiralty accepted the need to stock citrus fruits, its navy gained mastery over its French and Spanish rivals. Lind had introduced the important scientific principle that experimental groups should differ only on exposure to the tested intervention, all other variation being random. Causation would thus be clear.

The randomised controlled trial was refined by statistician Ronald A Fisher, who supervised its application in agricultural experiments in the 1920s. Statistical techniques of the time were rather impractical for the real world, but through his experience in trials Fisher made the procedure for comparing groups more accessible. He devised analysis of variance, and resolved a flaw in Pearson's correlational test by introducing the concept of degrees of freedom. In a publicised demonstation of experimental design, he tested whether a lady could distinguish by taste whether milk had been added to a cup before or after tea. To avoid bias, Fisher urged blinding of both subject and observer. Guided by his book *The Design of Experiments*, published in 1935, the randomised controlled trial became the standard method for pharmaceutical trials, and the model rapidly spread to other forms of treatment.

Meanwhile, the attention of psychiatry was drawn to the deterministic science of behaviourism. A leading figure was BF Skinner, whose experiments on operant conditioning demonstrated that human beings, like all other organisms, adhered to natural laws. Behaviourists offered potential prediction and manipulation of human behaviour, but the pursuit of a uniform set of behavioural variables was not fulfilled. Their procedures proved unsuitable for the study of complex human and social phenomena, which defied the precise delineation required for experimental study. Simplistic stimulus-response mechanisms and denial of free will were at odds with a growing revolutionary spirit in society. However, behavioural research had much influence on psychiatry, reinforcing the need for objective measurement and statistical precision. Token economy programmes were introduced in many a mental hospital ward. Clinical psychologists rose in stature as their behaviour modification techniques were their first direct contribution to treatment, adding to their skills in assessment and statistics.

Experimental design and rigorous statistical methodology were rapidly instilled in medicine in response to fatal flaws in treatment evaluation, as exposed by the lobotomy *debacle*. Science and ethics required higher standards of research, whether in laboratory or in practice. Authorship of psychiatric papers now typically included a statistician or psychologist versed in quantitative analysis, and tables and graphs proliferated. By the end of the 1950s, the literature of psychiatry was transformed. Paradoxically, the ascent of science encouraged a renewal of interest in traditional beliefs about madness.

Investigations begin

The 'search for lunacy' began in Kentucky, for that was the title and setting of the first systematic study of the Moon in psychiatry, published in the *Journal of Nervous and Mental Disease* in 1961.[2] The researcher was a psychologist, Loren Chapman, who persuaded the National Institute of Mental Health to fund the project. He designed the study in two parts, examining admissions and violence. He set two time divisions for lunar months: equal quarters of approximately eight days, and periods of three days around the exact time of new, full and half moons. Of 3,231 admissions at the Cook County Hospital assessment unit over a five-month period in 1957, the number admitted in each lunar period is shown below:

2   Chapman LJ (1961): 'A search for lunacy'. *Journal of Nervous and Mental Disease*, 132: 171–174.

Table 5.1 Psychiatric admissions (Chapman, 1961)

Moon phase	Mean admissions per day
New moon to first quarter	20.4
First quarter to full moon	23.1
Full moon to last quarter	20.5
Last quarter to new moon	22.3
New moon (+/-1 day)	18.8
First quarter (+/-1 day)	21.1
Full moon (+/-1 day)	21.2
Last quarter (+/-1 day)	21.8
Overall	21.7

Chapman applied Pearson's chi-square test to check for differences between actual and expected values. To reject the null hypothesis, the probability of an effect being due to chance should be less than one in twenty ($P = 0.05$). This is the conventional level of statistical significance. No lunar effect appeared, but Chapman acknowledged that admission was not the ideal variable as time often elapses between onset of disturbance and entry to hospital. He thought that a more conclusive answer to the lunacy question would be in measuring behaviour in the hospital. Clinical notes of three groups of patients were reviewed for incidents of violence, a behaviour traditionally linked to the Moon, and for which reliable records would be expected. At a veterans' administration hospital in Lexington, Chapman studied forty-one patients with schizophrenia, and thirty-nine described as 'paretics' (patients with the syphilitic condition, general paralysis of the insane). A third group comprised fifty-seven patients with chronic schizophrenia and a history of aggression at Chicago State Hospital. Reviewing individual records as far back as 1932, Chapman collated a total of 1,558 incidents. Again, no significant differences arose, although the peak in the three days around full moon could have been interesting if the study had been more numerically powered.

Table 5.2 Violent incidents with psychiatric patients (Chapman, 1961)

Phase	Schizophrenic group, Lexington	Paretic group, Lexington	Schizophrenic and violent group, Chicago	Total
New moon to first quarter	127	130	130	387
First quarter to full moon	160	131	126	417
Full moon to last quarter	151	115	125	391
Last quarter to new moon	131	113	119	363
New moon (+/-1 day)	40	41	61	142
First quarter (+/-1 day)	56	38	51	145
Full moon (+/-1 day)	75	49	67	191
Last quarter (+/-1 day)	48	57	58	163

Meanwhile, another study was conducted by Alex Pokorny, head of psychiatry and neurology at a veterans' administration hospital in Houston, Texas. Having explored various environmental factors in homicide and suicide, Pokorny had often heard references to the alleged provocative effects of the Moon. Obtaining data on all suicides and murders in Texas from 1959 to 1961, he tabulated the events by fortnightly periods around lunar phases, and did not find any lunar correlation (see below).[3]

---

3   Pokorny AD (1964): 'Moon phase, suicide and homicide'. *American Journal of Psychiatry*, 121: 66–67.

Table 5.3 Homicide and suicide, Texas (Pokorny, 1964)

Phase	Suicides	Homicides
New moon	1,251	1,012
Full moon	1,246	1,005
Apogee	1,251	1,024
Perigee	1,246	993
Total	2,497	2,017

Many readers would have concluded that the results from Chapman and Pokorny, the latter published in the world-leading *American Journal of Psychiatry*, had satisfactorily refuted the popular notion of lunar influence on behaviour. However, in the 1960s our satellite was constantly in the news, as the prime target of the space race. President Kennedy promised that before the decade was out, there would be a man (hopefully American) on the Moon. While many people looked up at the destined human conquest, others may have been spurred into thinking about what the Moon could do to us. Belief in its mischievous powers was common in the supposedly rational setting of the hospital.

Comments by emergency room doctors about an alleged full moon effect stimulated a study by psychiatrists Stephen Bauer and Edward Hornick.[4] Data on emergency visits to a psychiatric reception centre in the Bronx were collated for the 24-hour period of each phase, over two whole years from 1 January 1965. They found no real difference, a result replicated by another New York psychiatrist Diana Lilienfeld at a walk-in clinic. However, Bauer and Hornick conceded that if only a minority of psychiatric patients are influenced by the Moon, such effects might be lost in the data of a general sample.

---

4   Bauer SF, Hornick EJ (1968): 'Lunar effect on mental illness: the relationship of moon phase to psychiatric emergencies'. *American Journal of Psychiatry*, 125: 696–697.

Table 5.4 Emergency visits (Bauer and Hornick, 1968)

	Emergency visits	Mean proportion (%)
New moon	604	25.2
First quarter	588	24.5
Full moon	595	24.8
Last quarter	609	25.4

The first researcher to report a positive lunar result was Roger Osborn, a social worker in Ohio, who examined psychiatric admissions over the year 1965. He devised a strategy of time lagging, to allow for patients being admitted some days after initial mental disturbance. Although Osborn found a small but insignificant increase on the day of full moon, the correlation was strongest when the period was extended by four days. The paper was only accepted by a relatively obscure nursing journal, and its results were not supported by a similar study by Pokorny of admissions over a three-year period at a veterans' administration hospital. Applying the same time lag, Pokorny found a small but statistically significant excess at full moon in only one of three years — hardly a convincing result.

The Moon gave an unimpressive performance in the initial flurry of studies in the 1960s, but it took centre stage over in Miami, where a psychiatrist emerged as the leading advocate of the lunar hypothesis. Arnold Lieber, on beginning a psychiatric residency at Jackson Memorial Hospital, pursued a phenomenon observed both by himself during medical training, and by general hospital interns, whereby various symptoms such as epileptic seizures, psychological symptoms and bleeding from skin ulcers seemed to occur more frequently at full moon. All research projects required the sanction of the chairman of the university medical school, so Lieber knew that he would need to produce a scientifically sound proposal. After learning from meteorologists about the impact of the Moon on atmospheric tides, Lieber developed a hypothetical mechanism for lunar periodicity in behaviour: 'The Moon, via the effects of gravitational forces on the human organism, causes cyclic changes in water flow among the fluid compartments of the body.'[5] Biological tides, he speculated, were the result of the same force governing the ebb and flow of the seas. Related

5   Lieber AL, Sherin CR (1972): 'Homicides and the lunar cycle: toward a theory of lunar influence on human emotional disturbance'. *American Journal of Psychiatry*, 129: 69–74.

fluctuation in brain chemistry would be enough, in some people, to provoke irritability and emotional distress. The idea was not entirely eccentric: in a US government report *Biological Rhythms in Psychiatry and Medicine*, published in 1970, editor GG Luce considered human beings as 'cosmic receivers'.[6] The chairman was supportive, and even provided some preliminary funding.

Lieber engaged the statistical support of psychologist Carolyn Sherin, and they chose homicide as the event of interest. Unlike Pokorny, they restricted their study to events with a known date of injury, which was often some days before death. Records of all murders from two geographically distant counties were gathered: Dade in Florida, and Cuyahoga in Ohio, from the late 1950s to 1970. The 1,887 homicides in Dade County showed a remarkable peak at full moon, followed by a fall before rising again just after new moon. At full moon, there were eighty-five murders per day compared to the overall daily rate of sixty-three. Examining the cases, Lieber observed a disproportionately high number of events that were apparently completely irrational and out of character. In the concurrent data from Cuyahoga, a similar pattern appeared about three days later in the cycle, although this was not statistically significant. Apogee and perigee, to Lieber's surprise, did not show any effect at either location. The tentative conclusion was that biological tides produce changes in behaviour, with timing and magnitude altered by latitude. The results were announced at a symposium on chronobiology at Little Rock in 1971, and published in the *American Journal of Psychiatry* a year later, drawing much public interest – and professional scepticism. In correspondence with the journal, Lieber argued:

> More and more scientific evidence is being marshalled in support of the concept that man exists in dynamic equilibrium with his universe and may be more susceptible to the natural fluctuations of the cosmos than we have previously cared to admit.[7]

The next lunar report to appear in the prestigious pages of the *American Journal of Psychiatry* would be the last. Studying frequency of homicide in Houston, Alex Pokorny and Joseph Jachimczyk did not replicate Lieber's findings. Lieber later criticised their use of date of death; although 85 per cent of the deaths occurred within an hour of assault, the 15 per cent error was entirely in one direction (death always follows injury), producing bias. However, Pokorny and Jachimczyk felt sufficiently confident to assert that 'the effect of moon phases on homicide, suicide and mental ill-

6　Luce GG (ed, 1970): *Biological Rhythms in Psychiatry and Medicine*. Washington DC: United States Government Printing Office.

7　Lieber AL (1974): 'Comments on "Homicides and the lunar cycle" (reply)'. *American Journal of Psychiatry*, 131: 230.

ness should be viewed as a myth'.[8] In 1975, the journal published a letter urging the official journal of the American Psychiatric Association not to give further credence to a 'ludicrous issue'.[9] Earlier that year, 186 scientists, including physicians, astrophysicists and nineteen Nobel laureates, had signed a manifesto rejecting any recognition of astrology as a valid system.[10] Occult phenomena had no place in the serious scientific endeavour to which psychiatry pretended.

Underlying this reaction, psychiatry in the 1970s was very much on the defensive. Its claimed status as a scientific discipline was challenged by staunch critics from within (most notably RD Laing and Thomas Szasz) and from without. In 1973 American psychologist David Rosenhan produced an explosive paper *On Being Sane in Insane Places*, which seriously undermined public confidence in psychiatric diagnosis.[11] Rosenhan described the experiences of a group of pseudo-patients who got themselves admitted to various psychiatric hospitals after stating that they repeatedly heard the word 'thud' in their minds. Almost all were diagnosed as schizophrenic. Despite behaving normally throughout their stay, their activities were pathologised in the nurses' notes, with entries such as 'Patient engages in writing behaviour'. Most of the group were discharged as paranoid schizophrenics in remission. One hospital contacted Rosenhan, refusing to believe the same errors could be committed by their clinicians. A further group of fake schizophrenics was promised over a fixed period, and records revealed that of 193 admissions, 41 cases were suspected. In fact, Rosenhan had sent no patients. Meanwhile, evidence appearing in psychiatric journals revealed wide variation in diagnostic patterns not only between countries, but between hospitals in the same city. Clearly psychiatric assessment was not as scientific as purported. Even more shattering for professional prestige was the cinematic success of *One Flew over the Cuckoo's Nest*, which portrayed an oppressive regime in which the dreaded electroconvulsive therapy (ECT) was an instrument of discipline. Psychiatry was in dire need of justification, and trivialising reports on lunar influence threatened further detraction from its credibility.

Papers on lunar influence were confined to less conspicuous outlets, but a steady stream continued throughout the 1970s, providing evidence for and against the hypothesis.

Lieber persevered with his research, presenting further evidence in the lesser medium of the *Journal of Clinical Psychiatry* in 1978. Aware that cer-

8   Pokorny AD, Jachimczyk J (1974): 'The questionable relationship between homicides and the lunar cycle'. *American Journal of Psychiatry*, 131: 827–829, p828.

9   Levy NB (1975): 'On the Journal and the Moon'. *American Journal of Psychiatry*, 132: 85.

10   This had little effect, judging by a Gallup poll showing that belief in astrology among young Americans rose from 40 per cent in 1978 to 55 per cent in 1984.

11   Rosehan DL (1982): 'On being sane in insane places'. In *Social Research Ethics* (ed. M Bulmer). New York: Holmes & Meier, 15–37.

tain cosmic cycles were due to coincide in January 1974, Lieber had prepared to measure the impact on homicides and psychiatric crises. During
this time the Sun, Moon and Earth would be in syzygy (perfect alignment),
with gravitational pull maximised by perigee and perihelion. As expected,
there were extremely high tides, and with much anticipation Lieber
awaited data from his 'listening posts' at the psychiatric emergency room
at Jackson Memorial Hospital, the Dade County Medical Examiner, and
Miami Police Department. Assaults, fatal road accidents and psychiatric
emergencies increased, but not suicides. Meanwhile, a sharp rise in mur-
der was reported in the media, which Lieber cited as further support for
his biological tides theory, which he explained at greater length in his book
The Lunar Effect: Biological Tides and Human Emotions.

Before Lieber's second paper was published, two other studies were
published on the Moon and deviant behaviour in the community. Psychologists Jodi Tasso and Elizabeth Miller, examining records at Cincinnatti,
Ohio, found a full moon correlation with all categories of violent crime
except homicide. The relationship was strongest in domestic violence. By
contrast, analysis of police arrest frequency in Illinois over a seven-year
period by Forbes and Lebo showed no connection with lunar cycles.

Table 5.5 Summary of studies (1960s and 1970s)

Behaviour	Researchers and location	Year published	Lunar correlation*
Psychiatric admissions	Chapman (Cook County Hospital, Kentucky)	1961	None
	Osborn (psychiatric unit, Ohio State University College of Medicine)	1968	Full moon
	Pokorny (VA hospital, Houston, Texas)	1968	None
	Bauer and Hornick (reception centre, Bronx, New York)	1968	None
	Lilienfeld (walk-in clinic, New York)	1969	None
	Blackman and Catalina (community mental health centre, Staten Island, NY)	1973	Period following full moon

Table 5.5 continued

Behaviour	Researchers and location	Year published	Lunar correlation*
Psychiatric admissions	Walters, Markley and Tiffany (community mental health centre, Kansas)	1975	None
	Weiskott and Tipton (Austin State Hospital, Texas)	1975	Full moon and last quarter
	Geller and Shannon (Toronto)	1976	Full moon
	Climent and Plutchik (San Isidro Hospital, Cali, Colombia)	1977	New moon
Behavioural disturbance in psychiatric hospital	Chapman (VA hospital, Kentucky; Chicago State Hospital)	1961	None
	Shapiro, Streiner, Gray, Williams and Soble (Hamilton, Canada)	1970	None
Community telephone contacts	De Voge and Mikawa (crisis intervention service, Nevada)	1977	New moon
	Weiskott (counselling service for students, Austin, Texas)	1974	Fortnight of new moon
	Michelson, Wilson and Michelson (crisis service, Fort Lauderdale, Florida)	1979	None
Suicide	Pokorny (Texas)	1964	None
	Lester, Brockop and Priebe	1969	None
	Garth and Lester	1978	None
	Jones and Jones	1977	New moon
	Lieber (Dade County, Florida)	1978	None

Table 5.5 continued

Behaviour	Researchers and location	Year published	Lunar correlation*
Parasuicide and self-harm	Taylor and Diespecker (New South Wales)	1972	In females only, first quarter
	Ossenkopp and Ossenkopp (Winnipeg, Canada)	1973	In females only, apogee and perigee
Homicide and other crime	Pokorny (Texas)	1964	None
	Lieber and Sherin (Dade County, Florida; Cuyahoga County, Ohio)	1972	Full moon: homicide in Dade County only
	Pokorny and Jachimczyk (Harris County, Texas)	1974	None
	Tasso and Miller (Cincinnati, Ohio)	1976	Full moon: all crimes (rape, assault, burglary, theft, domestic violence) except murder
	Forbes and Leno	1977	None
	Lieber (Dade County, Florida)	1978	Full moon: homicides, assaults; new moon: first quarter
	Frey, Rotton and Barry	1979	None

* only included if statistically significant

The black, white and grey

By the end of the decade, a multitude of studies on lunar influence had appeared in the literature, as shown above. To make sense of the contradictory results, Kansas psychologists David Campbell and John Beets conducted a review. Their paper, published in *Psychological Bulletin* in 1978, criticised the importance given to statistically significant but spurious differences. As they explained, the probability (*P*) level of 0.05 is not suitable for multiple comparisons, because evidence of a real effect is diluted with each test. The more times the same data are analysed, the higher the likelihood of a chance correlation. According to Campbell and Beets, the output of studies was riddled with such false positives, known as Type I statistical error. Indeed, they accused researchers of 'massaging' their data until something interesting emerged. Apparent lunar periodicity could have resulted from other temporal effects, such as acknowledged by Weiskott, who attributed correlation of full moon and admissions to insurance renewals at the end of the month. Incidents such as violent crime and visits to A & E (accident and emergency) departments are known to increase at weekends, and a study of lunar influence would either need to control for this effect, or be of sufficient duration to negate this factor. Campbell and Beets also highlighted publication bias, with positive results more likely to reach print. They concluded that 'the general failure of the studies reviewed here to find a relationship between lunar phase and human behavior should be sufficient to discourage future investigators from further examining the lunar hypothesis'.[12]

In 1982, the journal *Environment and Behavior* hosted a debate on lunar influence. The case for lunacy was put by Salvatore Garzino, a social scientist who had introduced an innovative course on 'body time and human behaviour' in Tempe, Arizona. Reviewing eighteen published studies, Garzino found plenty of support for lunar influence. He noted that Campbell and Beets had omitted some positive reports from their review, including the findings suggestive of a gravitational effect by Klaus-Peter and Margitta Ossenkopp. By contrast to Campbell and Beets, he suspected Type II error, a failure to reject the null hypothesis due to inadequate statistical power. Pokorny's study of admissions, for example, had shown a full moon excess in each of the three years, but in two of the years the prob-

---

12   Campbell DE, Beets JL (1978): 'Lunacy and the moon'. *Psychological Bulletin*, 85: 1123–1129, p1127.

ability of error was slightly over 0.05. The debate highlighted the limitations of P values in scientific evaluation. Statistical significance is dichotomous: either a result reaches a desired threshold or not; the strength or importance of a relationship between variables is not shown. The larger the sample, the smaller the effect-size needed to reach the level of significance. Consequently, Campbell and Beets had asserted that evidence of an effect in smaller samples would be more persuasive. However, as lunar influence is likely to be weak overall, Garzino argued that its detection requires large-scale studies. By paradox, reducing the likelihood of Type I error increases the risk of Type II error, and vice versa. Suggesting that lunar periodicity may have been obscured by inconsistency in design and excessively broad classification of behaviours; Garzino emphasised that research on such complex phenomena remained at a primitive stage, lacking clear explanatory, outcome and confounding variables.

Garzino having supported in principle Lieber's view of the Moon as one of several regulators of body rhythms, David Campbell took the opportunity to respond (by quirk, at time of publication the tenures of himself and his opponent had converged on Humboldt State University in California). Campbell argued that in supporting time lagging and other procedures, Garzino had accepted positive results from a wide range of time intervals. Indeed, there were almost as many time divisions as studies. Some researchers had defined full moon as the day of its occurrence, others as the middle point of three days, a week or a fortnight, and still others as the period until the last quarter or new moon. It seemed theoretically dubious that a lunar effect appeared at full moon in one study location and at new moon in another. Campbell dismissed the biological tides theory on the basis that terrestrial gravity overwhelms the relatively light force exerted by the Moon, and argued that other putative mechanisms discussed by Garzino, such as fluctuations in atmospheric ions, would be of negligible influence at most.

The review of evidence by Campbell and Beets was of the traditional type: descriptive, of narrative flow, and with qualitative conclusions. In the 1980s the systematic method of meta-analysis was established, whereby the value of multiple, typically small-scale studies is maximised by synthesising the results. In a paper in 1980, Donald Templer and David Veleber, psychologists in California, combined data from published studies in an effort to produce an overall estimate of a lunar effect on mental disturbance. They collated the results of studies that had either divided the lunar month into equal periods (the most common approach), or applied a three-day period around new and full moon. For the former analysis, seven published studies were included, plus two new studies by the authors on telephone contacts and hospital admissions. No differences appeared between lunar quarters. However, when Templer and Veleber removed the contribution of Forbes and Leno, which had accounted for 76 per cent of the total data, a statistically significant elevation occurred in last quarter. In their analysis of results from three-day periods, which was limited to two previously published studies and the authors' own data, events peaked at new moon.

Aggregating results from independent studies reduces the effect of chance and local confounding factors, but considerable difficulties arise from the inconsistent methods and quality of studies. The criteria set by Templer and Veleber excluded the majority of published studies, and they only used published data. A more thorough meta-analysis was performed by psychologists James Rotton of Florida International University, and Ivan Kelly of the University of Saskatchewan, which appeared in a paper extending to twenty-one pages in *Psychological Bulletin* in 1985. Regarding the issue as primarily statistical, they gathered the results of every published study since 1961. Instead of simply analysing the reported results, Rotton and Kelly obtained data sets from Lieber, Pokorny, Forbes, Frey and Tasso, thus limiting publication bias. It was possible to repeat or at least scrutinise the analysis in twenty-three of the total of thirty-seven studies, and Rotton and Kelly found technical and computational errors in ten of these. Statistically naïve researchers had misapplied the chi-square test for significance; this procedure requires each datum to be fully independent, but a lunar effect would present a serial dependency. A few studies had used linear regression, thus showing the strength and direction of relationship between continuous numerical variables (e.g., frequency of behaviour/fraction of lunar surface illuminated), but only one study (by Michelson, Wilson and Michelson in 1979) had used the more appropriate method of time series analysis.

Fourier transformation (named after the nineteenth century French mathematician) is a method of time series analysis that detects hidden trends in longitudinal data, after taking account of known variability. Temporal patterns are displayed as a sine wave, a mathematical function describing a smooth, repetitive oscillation in data. To illustrate, A & E visits have a weekly cycle (with a weekend peak), seasonal patterns and annual effects (e.g., Christmas). Once these predictable factors have been controlled, residual variation will appear, some of which may be readily explained (e.g., drunken and disorderly behaviour increases during major sporting events such as the World Cup). Applying the Fourier transformation, Michelson, Wilson and Michelson found four periodicities in their eight years of data on crisis calls, lasting 7, 18, 35 and 76 days. None of these matched lunar cycles. Although time series analysis has become a common technique for lunar research since the 1980s, studying heterogenous groups may mask cyclicity in an unidentified group of susceptible people.

While acknowledging that Lieber had shown a small, insignificant increase in criminal behaviour at full moon, overall Rotton and Kelly found little evidence of correlation with synodic or anomalistic lunar cycles, nor did there appear a latitudinal relationship, as claimed by Lieber. Even if positive results were accepted, the effect was too miniscule for predictive value. Dissuading students from wasteful endeavour, Rotton and Kelly asserted: 'Just as we cannot prove that werewolves, unicorns and other interesting creatures do not exist, we cannot prove that the Moon does not influence behaviour.'[13] The Moon might have some as yet unknown powers over the mind, but the burden of proof was with the believers. Rotton and Kelly also presented their findings in *Skeptical Inquirer*, the periodical of the Committee for the Scientific Investigation of Claims of the Paranormal, a body of positivist scientists including BF Skinner, which in 1984 had persuaded American newspapers to carry a disclaimer for their astrology columns.[14]

Two years later, a further critique was presented by psychologists JJ Cyr and RA Kalpin, from Whitby Psychiatric Hospital in Ontario. They remarked on the ad hoc status of lunacy research, and a tendency for researchers to extrapolate findings from a single study setting to support or refute the whole lunacy hypothesis, rather than constraining their conclusions to the context studied. They disagreed with the statistical doctrine of Rotton and Kelly, seeing the fundamental problem in design rather than in data analysis. According to Cyr and Kalpin, reviewers had misrepresented replication, the bedrock of scientific validation, which should entail applying an identical study procedure on a different sample. The only researcher to have attempted this was Pokorny, who followed Osborn's study of admissions in 1968, but even here, inclusion criteria and delineation of lunar periods were not matched. Instead of studying periodicity in broad diagnostic categories and events, Cyr and Kalpin urged researchers to take a step back, and to undertake developmental work on specification of behavioural variables, which could then be tested for validity and reliability. Robustly designed exploratory studies would be amenable to replication, facilitating a systematic, generalisable evidence base on which the lunacy hypothesis could be properly assessed.

Rotton and Kelly, aided by physicist-mathematician Roger Culver, were not impressed by this proposed programme. With their increasingly scathing responses to studies reporting lunar correlation, they went on the offensive against what they regarded as a distortion of science. Their scorn did nothing to discourage Arnold Lieber from issuing a revised edition of

---

13   Rotton J, Kelly IW (1985a): 'Much ado about the full moon: a meta-analysis of lunar-lunacy research'. *Psychological Bulletin*, 97: 286–306.

14   Another prominent member was scientist Carl Sagan, who was a believer in lunar influence on human beings.

his book, retitled *How the Moon Affects You*, and lunar research has continued to appear in peer-reviewed journals. In the 1980s and 1990s the American bimonthly *Psychological Reports* published several studies, both
supporting and refuting the hypothesis. In its policy statement this journal
welcomes speculative and controversial articles; among the offerings in an
edition randomly selected from my university's library (December 1989)
were studies titled 'Changes in humor appreciation of college students in
the last 25 years'; 'The relation between competitive experience in
mid-childhood and achievement motives among male wrestlers'; and
'Some *Crocodile Dundee* after-effects in Northern Australia'. Papers on
lunar influence have also appeared in specialist journals on affective disorder, epilepsy, emergency medicine, cardiovascular disease, fertility,
gastro-intestinal disorders and sleep. As shown in Table 9 below, the
theme of contradictory findings persists. Every year, more studies appear.
What can we conclude from this smorgasbord of evidence? In the second
half of this book, the theory and evidence will be explored in greater depth
to explain the persistent belief — and disbelief — in the power of Moon on
mind.

Table 5.6 Recent studies (selected)

Condition / event	Study results	
	Lunar correlation	**No lunar correlation**
Suicide	Partonen *et alia* (Finland, 2004): excess at new moon	Voracek *et alia* (2008): all suicides in Austria, 1970–2006
Self-poisoning	Toofani and Musavi (Iran, 2001): excess in days around full moon	Rogers, Masterton and McGuire (1991): insignificant lunar cyclicity at poisoning centre, Edinburgh
Crisis calls	Kollerstrom and Steffert (UK, 2003): increase in calls by women at new moon, while calls by men decreased	Wilson and Tobacyk (Louisiana, 1989): 1% of variance explained by Moon, authors saw as 'negligible'
Behavioural disturbance in hospital/care home	Hicks-Casey and Potter (Tennessee, 1991): full moon excess in women with severe learning difficulties	Owen *et alia* (Sydney, 1998): aggressive incidents in five acute units
Psychiatric patients in the community	Barr (UK, 2000): full moon effect in schizophrenia, not in other conditions	Amaddeo *et alia* (Italy, 1997): no impact on frequency of contact with psychiatric services in South Verona
General practice consultations	Neal and Colledge (UK, 2000): anxiety and depression in sixty practices; peak six days after full moon	Wilkinson *et alia* (1997): records of a London practice, 1971–1988
Violence in community	Biermann *et alia* (Bavaria, 2009): no overall correlation, but excess of outdoor crime at full moon	Nunez *et alia* (2002): victims at A & E unit in Tenerife
Epileptic seizures	Polychronopoulus *et alia* (Greece, 2006): clustering at full moon at epilepsy emergency clinic	Benbadis *et alia* (2004): no effect; however, full moon peak in non-epileptic seizures

Six

Our mischievous minds

When historian of science George Sarton sailed on *Lady Drake* to the Windward Islands in 1936, he visited Fort Charlotte on Berkshire Hill, an old military fort converted into an institution for the poor. Part of the structure was used as a mental asylum, and Sarton was informed by a guard that the inmates were usually manageable, but required extra restraints at full moon. Sarton did not dispute the temporal association, but attributed this to patients reacting to oppressive measures, their agitation and aggression reinforcing the staff delusion. However, Sarton counselled against outright dismissal of a relationship between Moon and mind, arguing that some unknown effect was not inconceivable: 'The superstition lies not in the concept but in taking it for granted without warrant.'[1]

Often the motive for conducting studies on lunar influence was to scrutinise and potentially disprove what the researchers considered to be a figment of collective imagination. Psychiatrists Bauer and Hornick described the background for their investigation of lunar influence on psychiatric emergencies:

> As part of our interest in the structure and function of a psychiatric emergency service in a large municipal general hospital we noted repeated comments on the part of psychiatric staff about the effects of the moon on the frequency of use of the emergency service. Typically, after a particularly busy shift a psychiatric resident would suggest that there was really some connection between his busy tour of duty and the full moon of the previous night.[2]

Shapiro and colleagues, reporting on their study of mental hospital patients' notes, justified their attention to a dubious idea:

> While as a scientist it is easy to lean back in a swivel chair and make paternalistic disparaging remarks about such associations of psychopathology and the moon, it is a commonly accepted belief among nurses, aides, and attendants in mental health settings that the

---

1   Sarton G (1939): 'Lunar influences on living things'. *Isis*, 30: 495–507.
2   Bauer and Hornick (1968), p696.

patients 'act out' more during a full moon ... There are staff members who regularly arrange that their days off coincide with a full moon.[3]

The extent of lunar belief

For the case against lunar influence, it seems inconvenient that the believers are not 'lesser-spotted' freaks but the 'common or garden' operatives of public services. Several surveys have been conducted on the prevalence of lunar belief among psychiatric personnel, students and the general public. Dingman, Cleland and Swartz reported in 1970 that 4 per cent of attendants in a mental institution spontaneously mentioned the full moon as a cause of behavioural disturbance among patients. MD Angus, in an unpublished thesis at Simon Fraser University in British Columbia in 1973, found high prevalence of lunacy belief among psychiatric nurses (sixty-four out of eighty-six), yet recording of behavioural disturbance did not differ between believers and disbelievers; a full moon effect could not be discerned from the ward notes. From a single item in a survey of paranormal beliefs in psychology students at a Canadian university, GW Russell and M Dua in 1983 found that 45 per cent of 402 respondents believed that the Moon affected human behaviour. In 1984, LP Otis and ECY Kuo reported similar results among students in Canada and Singapore. If lunacy is all in the mind, the grey matter of the bright young things appeared as prone as that of long-in-the-tooth nurses.

Although several standardised instruments for assessing occult beliefs existed, none was specifically related to the Moon. In 1985, James Rotton and Ivan Kelly, authors of the aforementioned meta-analysis, devised the Belief in Lunar Effects Scale (BILE), with the following dichotomous statements:[4]

1 lunar phases play an important role in human affairs;

2 there is some truth to the idea that 'crazies' come out when the moon is full;

3 some people behave strangely when the moon is full;

4 I have never felt that the moon affects my behaviour;

5 it is a good idea to stay at home when the moon is full;

6 my own behaviour is affected by phases of the moon;

7 a full moon can trigger violence and aggression;

---

3   Shapiro *et alia* (1970), pp827–828.
4   Rotton J, Kelly IW (1985b): 'A scale for assessing belief in lunar effects: reliability and concurrent validity'. *Psychological Reports*, 57: 239–245.

8 there is absolutely no relationship between phases of the moon and behaviour;

9 only superstitious people believe that a full moon influences behaviour.

The scale was subjected to the usual psychometric tests for reliability and validity, and normative data was produced from a sample of 157 undergraduate students. Older respondents were more likely to believe in lunar influence. There were no differences by gender, education, social class or religious affiliation, but higher scores were found in regular churchgoers. Those believing in lunar effects made most errors in a logic test, comprising a set of categorical syllogisms. However, the example provided by the authors shows the problem of applying axiomatic logic, rather than the doubting attitude of the true scientist, to mysterious phenomena: 'If flying saucers really existed, somebody would have photographed them. Nobody has ever photographed a flying saucer. Therefore, flying saucers do not exist.'

The BILE scale was then tested on groups known to harbour lunar beliefs, to check whether differences could be detected. This is another standard developmental procedure for rating scales. Mental health workers and police officers were approached, as well as randomly selected members of the public interviewed on beaches or park benches. A significantly higher rate of lunar beliefs was found in the police than in the other groups. The mental health sample, in which all doctors were male and all nurses female, produced only slightly higher scores than the passers-by. The authors contrasted an unintellectual police culture with the enlightening effect of scientific literature in health practitioners. For Rotton and Kelly, lunar belief was the product of ignorance, but the apparently superior rationale of pedestrians over police officers was not discussed in their concluding remarks.

Table 6.1 BILE scores (Rotton and Kelly, 1986)

Group	Respondents	Mean BILE score (SD*)
Mental health workers	36	9.61 (3.62)
Police officers	48	11.82 (3.72)
Pedestrians	60	8.97 (4.30)

*standard deviation

Physician Daniel Danzl used a modified version of the BILE scale at a department of emergency medicine in Kentucky. The sample comprised twenty-five nurses and the same number of physicians, with 80 per cent and 64 per cent respectively showing lunar belief. The author found such supernaturalism among professional colleagues difficult to comprehend. In a volley of sarcasm rarely found in the pages of a serious journal, Danzl proposed the following strategies for dealing with full moon in an emergency unit:[5]

1   Evaluate antilunium hydrochloride, containing physostigmine, ergotamine, lithium, benztropine, belladonna, phenobarbital, and a quadricyclic antidepressant. If effective, market as 'Eclipse moontabs'.

2   Pill configuration may trigger lunar overdoses. Since antipsychotics and antidepressants are round (full) or crescent-shaped (waxing/waning), repackage in tamper-proof cubettes.

3   In deference to the 'tidal theory', shelter moonstruck nephrotics, cirrhotics, and congestive heart failure victims.

4   Standardise the 'man in the moon' scale for lunar mental status examinations. Galileo's maria, which contain innumerable constellations of objects, are observed through a skylight that filters moonshine.

5   Establish 'lunar stress syndrome' as a defense in perilunar malpractice litigation.

6   In seasonal affective disorder, the darkness of winter triggers the pineal to secrete melatonin. Pursue isolation of a psychotropic hormone, lunatonin, secreted in moonlight.

7   Avoid scheduling moonlighters on lunar shifts. Never post lunar calendars, and remove moon pies from vending machines in waiting rooms.

8   Emergency department moon-music or looney tune selection should avoid thought insertion cuts like the *Brain Damage* lyrics 'The lunatic is in my head' on Pink Floyd's *Dark Side of the Moon.*

In the *Journal of Social Psychology* in 1989, behavioural scientists James Wilson and Jerome Tobacyk of Louisiana Technical University assessed lunar belief at a mental health telephone crisis centre. Firstly, they examined the frequency of crisis calls, and found that slightly under 1 per cent of variation was of lunar timing (although they erroneously demarcated the cycle as a period of twenty-eight days). Secondly, they used the BILE scale to test their hypothesis that crisis centre staff would have a higher rate of belief than a comparative group of university students. Their *t*-test confirmed a statistically significant difference, and a regression model showed that although the crisis workers were older, age was not a significant factor.

5   Danzl DF (1987): Lunacy. *Journal of Emergency Medicine,* 5: 91-95.

Table 6.2 Lunar beliefs in crisis workers and students (Wilson and Tobacyk)

	Respondents	Mean age (SD*)	Mean BILE score (SD*)
Crisis workers	87	37.7 (14.9)	26.8 (8.1)
Students	102	21.1 (5.5)	22.3 (7.8)

* standard deviation

David Vance (1995) at University of New Orleans surveyed various beliefs of 325 adults from the general population in Kentucky, including two items on lunar effects: 'I think the moon makes some people act weird or crazy'; and 'I believe people act up during full moons'.[6] Overall, 140 respondents (43 per cent) answered positively to one or both of the statements. There was no correlation with age, sex or education, but occupational differences emerged. The rather flimsy report did not include statistical testing of differences between the eight categories of occupation, but it was interesting that lunar beliefs were proportionately highest in the twenty-six mental health practitioners (twenty-one; 81 per cent) and lowest in students (twenty-two of ninety-two; 24 per cent). Overall, from the results of surveys it may be concluded that while common in the public at large, belief in the powers of the Moon are relatively pervasive in the setting of mental health care. Why this persistence of occultism in a professional environment?

Psychological roots

One explanation for lunar belief is in locus of control, a concept devised by New York psychologist Julian Rotter (1916–). In the 1950s, when the gulf in psychology between psychodynamics and behaviourism was at its widest, Rotter launched his social learning theory, which emphasised the influence of the social environment on motives and expectations. In 1966 he produced a 13-item scale for differentiating internal and external locus of

6   Vance DE (1995): 'Belief in lunar effects on human behavior'. *Psychological Reports*, 76: 32–34.

control. People scoring highest believe that destiny is in their own hands; respondents with extremely low scores consider their fate to be inescapable. In a survey of 97 college students in 1981, Dale Jorgenson administered Rotter's scale and an unpublished Lunar Beliefs Inventory relating to 120 mental states and behaviours. As anticipated, students with external locus of control made the most positive associations with the Moon.

A related theory of how people make sense of their world is attribution theory, introduced by Viennese social psychologist Fritz Heider (1896–1988) in his book *The Psychology of Interpersonal Relations* in 1958. Heider noted how people act as amateur psychologists, inferring causes to their own and other people's behaviour. Where individual behaviour is in tune with the social setting, people tend to regard the situation as the stimulus, but if someone's behaviour deviates from norms, for whatever reason, it is attributed to individual disposition. Attributional tendencies are prone to bias, in that while others are considered to be predominantly influenced by their environment, people think of themselves as relatively autonomous. We may take credit for success, while blaming others for our failures. Faulty attribution in psychiatry was sensationally demonstrated in the 1970s by David Rosenhan's fake schizophrenic patients, indicating that once someone is diagnosed, all behaviour and characteristics are coloured by that label. The person, therefore, is no longer expressing the self but a disease process; all behaviour is attributed to a generalised condition rather than individual agency. As radical psychiatrist RD Laing stated, a 'schizophrenic' is simply someone who a psychiatrist considers to be schizophrenic. It could be argued that psychiatry, with its symptomatic tautology, is predicated on an attributional system.

Attribution theory is relevant to lunar belief because of social pressure to conform to prevailing attitudes, which are internalised by group members. The relationship of the Moon to mental derangement may be regularly reinforced in a mental health setting, such that new members are persuaded that there must be truth in the idea. Unlike Jorgensen, Rotton and Kelly claimed to have found no correlation between BILE scores and personality traits, but reported that while 49 per cent of respondents believed that the Moon might induce strange behaviour in other people, only 14 per cent thought that this was also true of themselves. Although not considered by the authors, this finding would suggest attributional bias.

The context of mental health nursing, particularly in the remote psychiatric institutions prior to community care, may have provided a fertile ground for lunar belief. As sociologists have described, nursing, despite its professional charter, continues to be regarded both by the public and within its own membership as a vocation rather than a profession. Historically, unlike the middle-class background of nurses in general hospitals, the nursing staff of the asylums was mostly drawn from the lower echelons of society. A career in the asylum was unappealing, with poor pay, long hours and punitive discipline. The work of the mental nurse was akin to that of a prison officer, locking and unlocking doors at every turn, and maintaining order on wards of up to a hundred inmates. For the minions of asylumdom, academic pursuits rarely continued beyond memorising the basic training manual for the mental nursing certificate. In an isolated culture, lay attitudes to madness prevailed, and ideas such as a full moon effect were probably accentuated by mental hospital lore. Several highly experienced nursing acquaintances of the author insist that a lunar effect was readily discernible in the wards of the old mental institutions. Charlie Russell, who practised over four decades at the former hospitals of Hartwood in Lanarkshire, and Cane Hill and Netherne in Surrey, recalled a consensus among colleagues that shifts were more hectic when the Moon was full.

Lunar belief may be an element of the psychological defences deployed by nurses to survive occupational adversity. In her classic observational research on nurses, published in 1960, Isobel Menzies described how self-serving routines reduce anxiety in an unpredictable environment. Her study focused on general nurses, but the findings were equally applicable to the daily routine of the mental hospital:

> Elaborate rituals have been devised in order to distance the nurse from the emotional life of the patient. Detachment from the job is achieved through routinisation of simple self-care tasks, and personal responsibility is taken out of the hands of those delivering care, thereby providing enough distance between the doer and the one who takes responsibility for all sorts of blame transference to take place.[7]

Mental health nursing had even stronger motives for defensive ritual, because of its stigma by association. As described by Erving Goffman in his sociological critique of the asylum, nurses drew boundaries between themselves and their deviant charges. Regarding patients but not themselves as prone to lunar influence perhaps demonstrates this tendency to enforce social distance. Concluding from their survey of mental health crisis staff, Wilson and Tobacyk suggested that the unpredictabilities of the job led workers to attribute behaviour to an external cause, thereby retaining a modicum of control. David Vance made a similar point in his paper. By inferring lunar causation, nurses denied the random volition that threatened stability, while also relinquishing themselves from responsibility for a disorderly shift.

Lunar belief was likely to be perpetuated by the cognitive bias of expectancy and selective recall. Although not measured by their study, Wilson and Tobacyk remarked on how beliefs might affect observations of activ-

7   Menzies IEP (1960): 'The functioning of social systems as a defence against anxiety: a report on a study of the nursing service of a general hospital'. *Human Relations*, 13: 95–121.

ity at full moon. However, it is possible that the crisis workers had evidence that their comparative group of students lacked.

If belief in the power of the Moon was so prevalent in mental hospitals, why was it given such short shrift in the literature of psychiatry? A contrast may be drawn between the scientism of psychiatry and the anecdotalism of nursing. Psychiatry built its professional expertise on a conceptualisation of mental disorder as distinct diagnostic entities transcending the idiosyncrasies of patients, whereas the nursing role has always been individualist, dealing with thoughts, feelings and behaviour rather than symptomatic generalisation. Research on lunar influence in mental health settings has almost entirely been conducted by psychiatrists and psychologists, but it was the nursing staff that had most intensive contact with patients, managing wards for twenty-four hours a day. If a lunar effect existed, mental hospital nurses would have been best placed to observe it. However, as remarked by historian of mental nursing Peter Nolan, the notes recorded on patients shift after shift, year upon year, received scant attention from medical staff. With nurses expected to describe rather than explain, daily entries were limited to brief, mundane accounts of patients' daily activities. Explanatory offerings of workers unversed in the scientific approach were unlikely to be taken seriously by their medical masters; to suggest a link between a patient's behaviour and a full moon to a busy medical officer on his rounds risked ridicule.

As well as unique occupational factors, nurses' beliefs about the Moon may be a reflection of wider society. Hans Eysenck and David Nias, in a book scrutinising astrological belief, published in 1982, argued that any lunar pattern in suicide or other mental disturbance at new or full moon was likely to be a self-fulfilling prophecy influenced by what people read in horoscopes. Eysenck (1916–1997), head of clinical psychology at the Maudsley Hospital in London from 1946 to 1983, was an arch empiricist much appreciated by psychiatrists for his debunking of psychoanalysis as a pseudoscience. His insistence on concrete fact alone as the basis of truth coloured his investigation of astral occultism. In a chapter devoted to the Moon, selective reporting abounds. However, the authors drew short of dismissing any possibility of lunar influence, Eysenck perhaps having learned from the controversy around his thesis on psychoanalysis, when he was portrayed as an absolutist too quick to dismiss theory for which adequately sensitive research methods had yet to be developed.[8] Eysenck softened his stance in later years, displaying a decidedely open mind in the book *Explaining the Unexplained*, written with Carl Sargent, an expert on paranormal activity. Here, Eysenck and Sargent berated scientists for rigidly adhering to their own unsound belief system, which was presented

8   For example, Harry Guntrip (1964): *Healing the Sick Mind*. London: George Allen & Unwin.

as a fallacious syllogism: there are known laws of nature; parapsychology does not follow these laws; therefore parapsychology must be untrue. The evidence for some cases of extrasensory perception had been sufficient to persuade an erstwhile cynic.

Faith and fantasy

Eric Chudler, in his chapter on the lunar legend in the volume *Tall Tales about the Mind and Brain: Separating Fact from Fiction,* attributed lunar belief to childhood exposure to popular fairy tales, of which he gave four examples.[9] *Goodnight Moon* by MW Brown (1947) and *Goodnight, Goodnight* by Eve Rice (1980) present the Moon as a prominent symbol of the night, with mystical imagery. In *Moongame* by Frank Asch (1984), during a game of hide-and-seek the Moon hides behind a cloud, to the consternation of his friend Bear. Maurice Sendak's *Where the Wild Things Are* (1963) tells the story of Max, who one evening dons a wolf costume and causes mischief, for which his mother sends him to bed without supper. In his room, a wild forest and sea emerges in his imagination, and Max sails to the land of the Wild Things. He conquers these scary monsters by staring into their yellow eyes without blinking, and is made king of the Wild Things. Max and the strange beasts dance and howl at the Moon, which appears on most pages of an evocatively illustrated book, and has been interpreted as the author's own mother from his strict Jewish upbringing in Brooklyn keeping eye on her rebellious but creative son. Over twenty million copies have been sold.

The Man in the Moon is an enduring idea, based on an apparent resemblance of the lunar disc to a human face, an image formed by the larger *Mare*. However, full and crescent moons are often embellished by artistic licence, depicted without reference to the actual features of the lunar surface. In legend, the Man in the Moon was in exile for theft; in the Roman version, having stolen one too many sheep. A traditional English verse makes mirth of the mystical lunar being:

> The man in the moon came down too soon,
> and asked his way to Norwich
> They sent him south and he burnt his mouth
> By eating cold pease-porridge.

9   Chudler EH (2007): 'The power of the full moon: running on empty?' In *Tall Tales about the Mind and Brain: Separating Fact from Fiction* (ed. S Dellasalla). Oxford: Oxford University Press, 401-410.

As well as its representation in fiction, the alluring Moon, with its benevolent glow and its dark side, has featured repeatedly in every genre of contemporary music from jazz to rock. The Moon is prominent in the verse and imagery of heavy metal bands, whose Satanic themes are probably more for shock value than black magic or worship of the Antichrist.[10] While the well known track *Dark Side of the Moon* by Pink Floyd is not really about the Moon, the idea reinforces the ancient theme of a Janos-faced orb. A direct reference to lunar caprice was made by the 1960s band Creedance Clearwater Revival:

> I see the bad moon rising
> I see trouble on the way
> I see earthquakes and lightning
> I see bad times today
> Don't go around tonight ...
> There's a bad moon on the rise

Apart from its role in fantasy, today the Moon has little significance in the West. However, in an increasingly multicultural society this may change. Islam maintains a lunar calendar and the Moon therefore is the marker of rituals such as Ramadan. The crescent moon is depicted on the flags of many Muslim nations, and while the pagan worship from which this symbol was probably derived was repudiated by Islam, the Moon often appears in love poetry, with the face of the beloved, accentuated by the headscarf, resembling the lunar disc.[11] The Koran has a chapter devoted to the Moon, Allah having gifted believers the monthly divisions of time. Perhaps taken more literally than in other monotheist religions, Islamic scripture maintains the doctrines of geocentrism and heavenly perfection. A case of indoctrination was described by popular astronomer Patrick Moore in response to a lunar eclipse in 1979, on which he had commented on television.[12] Schoolteachers in Bradford in Yorkshire were discussing the event on the following day in class. The town is home of a large Muslim population, and pupils who had attended five o'clock sermon at the mosque raised the objection that Islam forbade them from watching the event. Furthermore, some pupils had allegedly been told that the American landings on the Moon were propaganda and an insult to the heavenly domain. If true, such instruction was a departure from the spirit of the great Arab astronomers of the Middle Ages, and from the pro-

---

10   Asked by an interviewer whether Black Sabbath were advocates of black magic, lead singer Ozzy Osbourne replied: 'Are the Rolling Stones into avalanches?' (black-sabbath.com).

11   Mona Siddiqui, Islamic scholar at Glasgow University (personal communication).

12   Moore P (1992): *Fireside Astronomy*. Chichester: John Wiley & Sons.

nouncement of prophet Mohammed: 'He who travels in search of knowledge travels along Allah's path to paradise.'[13]

While the Moon has no specific powers in Islam, it has a more prominent role in eastern lands. Medical practice in the Indian subcontinent is strongly influenced by *ayurveda* (*ayur* and *veda* literally mean life and knowledge). This system is based on a model of vital energy, with similarities to Hippocratic medicine. Three factors are considered in the diagnosis and treatment of mental disorders: how food and drugs affect the mind; the extent of harmony between mind and body; and the relationship between mind and external world. Symptoms of chronic mental illnesses are believed to vary with lunar phases, particularly at the cusp of the full moon, and at 'black moon', when the moon is invisible.[14] The full moon is celebrated by Hindus in monthly 'purnima' festivals.

The autumn lunar festival, dating back to the moon worship of the Shang dynasty, is the second most important celebration of the Chinese calendar; people in the predominantly agricultural countries of the Orient sit outdoors at this time, eating 'moon cakes' and admiring the glowing orb. The strength of cultural belief about avoiding risk during the lunar festival was demonstrated by researchers Kuo, Coakley and Wood in 2010, with a marked decline in share turnover in east Asian stock markets. While reduced business activity during holiday periods is a global phenomenon, which Americans describe as 'gone fishing', the authors attributed a distinct effect to historically negative connotations with full moon.

The Judaeo-Christian heritage of the West is increasingly confronted by forces of change. Sociologist Peter Berger described how a rapid process of secularisation destroys cohesive networks and beliefs:

> As modern technological rationality penetrates a traditional society, the archaic unity of being is broken. The cosmic connection between all beings and all objects is severed. To the extent that componentiality extends even to the realm of social relations and to the individual's experience of himself, it tends to be experienced as uprooting and alienating.[15]

Yet alongside this agnosticism, the demographic flux of globalisation is rejuvenating the status of religion and traditional beliefs in Western society. Despite the rhetoric of intellectual celebrities such as Richard Dawkins and Stephen Fry, we may not be on a linear path to objective rationalism, but to a rather more interesting future of conflicting ideas about the meaning of our existence. Population statistics show a strong correlation

---

13 For more on the Moslem contribution to science see *Pathfinders: The Golden Age of Arabic Science* by Jim Al-Khalili of University of Surrey (2010). London: Allen Lane.
14 Shankar D, Unnikrishnan PM (ed. 2004): *Challenging the Indian Medical Heritage*. New Delhi: Foundation Books.
15 Berger PL, Berger B, Kellner H (1974): *The Homeless Mind: Modernization and Consciousness*. Harmondsworth: Penguin, pp133–134.

between religious fundamentalism and procreation, suggesting that teleology will outlive realist ontology.[16] In the internet era, people have access to a broad spectrum of ideas and knowledge, and make their own judgements about credibility. For example, despite attacks from the medical orthodoxy, 'alternative medicine', homeopathy, *Reiki* and acupuncture are flourishing. To learn about lunar influence on the mind, Google searchers are likely to seek sources that concord with their own outlook. Whether the Moon is regarded simply as a rock in space, as a metaphysical source of vitality, or as divine intervention, will be much influenced by the differential trends of sociodemography. From an anthropic perspective, the status of the Moon is continually evolving.

---

16   Report by Jonathan Leake, *Sunday Times* (2 January 2011): 'Atheists: a dying breed as nature favours faithful'.

Seven

A distracting glow

Of the many intellectual affiliations formed in the momentum of the Scientific Enlightenment, one name leaps out from the pages of history. Shaded in eminence only by the Royal Society, the Lunar Society of Birmingham had a distinguished membership including botanist and evolutionary theorist Erasmus Darwin (grandfather of Charles), chemist Joseph Priestley (who discovered oxygen), celebrated potter Josiah Wedgwood, and engineers James Watt and Matthew Boulton. It was so named because its gatherings in Birmingham were held on the nearest Monday to each full moon, enabling safe passage home in moonlight. The Lunar Society spent their evenings musing on steam power, canals and other grand schemes, thus laying the foundations of the Industrial Revolution. Some members were ideologically radical, supporting the French Revolution and American independence. Perhaps as an eighteenth-century expression of anti-intellectualism, the society was popularly known as 'The Lunatics'.

Primitive man feared night and darkness, and saw the Moon as a kindly beacon. Prior to municipal lighting, streets were deemed unsafe at night, darkness providing cover for real or imagined clandestine exploits. Moonlight was regarded as a traveller's friend, and the monthly floodlight enabled an early start to agricultural labour. However, the full moon was a double-edged sword. Mysticism of witches and werewolves aside, the nocturnal lamp exposed the quarry of highwaymen and burglars; a 'moonlighter', according to *Everyman's English Dictionary*, was an Irish night-raider. In a modern, artificially lit environment, most people are unaware of lunar phases, but the variation in radiance is much more noticeable in a rural setting. With the night hours bathed in a silvery light, the traditional lore of the shires can seem compelling, but do moonbeams really have any power over body and mind?

Disruption to the body clock

Sleep disturbance has long been recognised as a factor in mental disorder. Reputed figures of the early asylum period, such as Esquirol, acknowledged the impact of nocturnal provocation.

> It is true, that the insane are more agitated at the full of the moon, as they are also, at early dawn. But is it not the light of the moon that excites them, as that of day, in the morning? Does not this brightness produce, in their habitations, an effect of light, which frightens one, rejoices another, and agitates all?[1]

Forbes Winslow, in his treatise *Light: Its Influence on Life and Health*, also attributed the legend of lunacy to the luminary stimulus. Lieutenant-Colonel CJ Lodge Patch, medical superintendent of the Punjab Mental Hospital in the latter years of the British Raj, concurred with the belief of indigenous personnel that patients were noisier at full moon, which he likened to the directional barking of hyenas and jackals. Yet moonlight has been neglected in recent textbooks on environmental factors in mental disorder, despite its potential aggravation of restless minds. For example, a weighty volume *The Impact of the Environment on Psychiatric Disorder*, edited by leading British psychiatrist Hugh Freeman, omits any mention of the Moon.[2] The book did, however, include a chapter on seasonal effects.

Seasonal affective disorder, or the 'winter blues' has only recently been established as a psychiatric condition, first appearing in the third edition of the *Diagnostic and Statistical Manual of Mental Disorders (DSM-III)* in 1987, but the concept is not new. Seasonal patterns in mania and melancholia were recognised long ago by Hippocrates and by Roman physicians. Esquirol in 1825 described a Belgian patient who suffered from depressive episodes in three successive winters, each time remitting in spring. Seasonal affective disorder was defined as a specific type of depression caused by lack of acclimatisation to long periods of darkness, and is most common at high latitudes such as in Scandinavia, where midwinter days are limited to a few hours around noon. In Iceland, the word

1   Esquirol (1837/1845), p32.
2   Freeman H, Stansfield S (eds 2008): *The Impact of the Environment on Psychiatric Disorder*. London: Routledge.

skammdegistghunglyndi literally means short day, heavy mood. Seasonal affective disorder is not simply a psychological response to the cold and dark, but a physiological fault in the body clock.

Chronobiology, a gradually expanding field of biomedical research, is concerned with the multitude of regulatory feedback systems of the body, including various intracellular processes, neural and cardiac rhythms, the sleep-wake pattern, monthly menstrual cycle, and seasonal adjustment. Specialists Russell Foster at Oxford University and Till Roenneberg at the Ludwig Maximilians University commented: 'the increasing tendency to work at odds with biological time is having a marked impact on our health, exacerbating cardiovascular disease, cancer, obesity and mental health problems'.[3] Natural rhythms can be severely disrupted by working night shifts, and by use of caffeine, nicotine and other stimulants. Most rhythmic processes in the body appear to have endogenous timing, but annual and diurnal rhythms are cued by signals from the geophysical environment.

A trailblazing investigator of mammalian rhythms was Jürgen Aschoff (1913–1998), who conducted experimental research at a bunker built into the hillside hear the monastery and brewery of Andechs in Bavaria. For over twenty years, he studied cycles under manipulated conditions. Aschoff formulated the Circadian Rule, whereby animal activity increases with the intensity of continuous illumination. Light is the most important *zeitgeber* (phase-setting factor) of the circadian clock. The other known environmental cue is temperature, which also falls in the evening, but there may be other unknown exogenous factors. The deliberately imprecise term 'circadian', coined by Franz Halberg from the Latin *circa* (about) and *dies* (day), was based on laboratory evidence that daily rhythms run to a roughly 24-hour pattern without any environmental regulation. Holding temperature and light constant, Aschoff found that the physiological day of study subjects typically lengthened to around twenty-five hours, although in exceptional cases the perceived duration shifted to as much as forty hours. Emerging into the daylight a month later, some subjects thought that they had spent only three weeks underground.

Despite omnipresent artificial lighting, our circadian rhythm has solar entrainment, being synchronised with the natural length of day as this gradually changes throughout the year. Most people find it harder to get up on a dark winter morning, as they do so unassisted by the pineal gland. This tiny, flat structure, shaped like a pine cone (hence its name), is located in the epithalamus. After being speculated by Descartes as the bridge of

3   Foster RG, Roenneberg T (2008): 'Human responses to the geophysical daily, annual and lunar cycles'. *Current Biology*, 18 (R): 784–794.

body and soul, the pineal gland faded into physiological obscurity; but in recent decades a wide range of functions has been revealed, with implications for neurological and behavioural disorders. Back in 1906 Simpson and Galbraith observed that diurnal temperature rhythms are regulated by the light–dark cycle, and in the 1960s it was discovered that the body clock operated through the secretions of the hormone melatonin, synthesised from serotonin by the pineal gland. At onset of dusk, impulses are sent from the retina via the optic nerve to the suprachiasmatic nucleus of the hypothalamus, the seat of the body clock. Messages are then relayed to the pineal gland to release melatonin into the bloodstream, permeating every tissue of the body. As morning light appears, melatonin levels subside and serotonin gradually alerts us to a new day.

Recent research in human beings and other vertebrates has revealed that the photoreceptor mechanism involves not the image-forming rods and cones of the outer retina, but a third type of receptors. Sensitive ganglion cells in the inner retina provide the light detecting system for the dawn–dusk cycle. Blood levels normally reach a peak around two o'clock in the morning. As long-distance travellers know, the body clock can be temporarily offset by the rapid time-zone changes of air travel. Whereas jet lag has been successfully treated with melatonin supplements, the enduring condition of seasonal affective disorder is not so amenable to artificial hormone delivery. However, since the first clinical trial in 1981, phototherapy has been used to counter the depressive effect of long periods of darkness. The sleep–wake cycle is of solar synchronicity, but could other environmental stimuli offset the body clock? Swedish psychiatrist Lennart Wetterberg stated: 'Acute exposure to light at night reduces the nocturnal decline of core body temperature and inhibits the secretion of the pineal hormone melatonin.'[4]

As revealed by the equations of James Clerk Maxwell in 1973, visible light is a part of the spectrum of electromagnetic radiation. Its intensity is 250 times brighter at full moon than on a clear, starry night at new moon. Melatonin secretion can be suppressed by sufficiently bright light. A 1987 edition of *Science* journal presented a debate on whether moonlight was strong enough to influence the human circadian rhythm. While acknowledging that further research was necessary on a lunar effect, Harvard sleep specialist Charles Czeisler explained that the Moon is dwarfed by the power of artificial lighting. From a domiciliary perspective, a full moon is seventy times less powerful than a 100-watt lightbulb. Writing in *Nature* journal in 2002, California biologists Satchidananda Panda, John

4   Wetterburg L (1998): 'Melatonin in adult depression'. In *Melatonin in Psychiatric and Neoplastic Disorders* (eds M Shafii M, SL Shafii). American Psychiatric Press, 43–79.

Hogenesch and Steve Kay suggested that 'circadian photoreception may have evolved to use a separate mechanism and perhaps separate photoreceptors to filter out weak stimuli, such as lightning and moonlight, which would otherwise mimic light conditions such as dawn and dusk'.[5] Unlike electrical storms, lunar cycles are a consistent phenomenon to which the body clock of some species has adapted. Research on light stimulation, quantified in lux, does not indicate that the Moon would much impact on human physiology. According to professor of circadian neuroscience Russell Foster, even the starkest lunar glare is unlikely to suppress melatonin.[6]

Indoor lighting, however, has been shown to affect melatonin secretion and to shift the sleep–wake phase. Zeitzer, Czeisler and colleagues in 2000 administered varying levels of experimental light to twenty-three healthy volunteers, finding that the circadian rhythm is more sensitive than previously thought to photic stimulation. Israeli sleep specialists Yaron Dagan and Michal Eisenstein reported that people with sleep disorders are prone to disturbance by light of quite low intensity. It appears that phase entrainment can be offset by room light in the late evening, or by a visit to the toilet in the early hours of the morning. Indoors, the brightness of the Moon cannot match that achieved by the flick of a switch. Yet there is evidence that a full moon does affect duration and depth of sleep. In 2006 Martin Röösli and colleagues at the University of Berne conducted a study in which thirty-one healthy volunteers completed sleep diaries for six weeks. Prospective self-reporting would have been prone to expectancy bias, but participants were only informed of the main objective of the research, which was to assess the impact of a nearby mobile telephone base station. Lunar phases were analysed as a continuous cosine function, with other variables controlled. Duration of sleep was an average of nineteen minutes less at full moon that at new moon (six hours and forty-one minutes compared to exactly seven hours). The paper was fittingly embellished with a title taken from a John Lennon and Yoko Ono song: 'Sleepless night, the Moon is bright'. The Bernese team did not believe that such difference would have psychiatric implications, but their findings were from the general population. Could the sleep differential be wider, with greater impact, in particular psychiatric or neurological conditions?

5   Panda S, Hogenesch JB, Kay SA (2002): 'Circadian rhythms from flies to human'. *Nature*, 417: 329–335.
6   Personal communication.

Full moon and mood disorder

Awareness is heightened in mania. Just as depression increases during winter gloom, the abundance of light in spring can cause restlessness and lead to a manic episode. Although insomnia tends to be regarded as a sequel to mental disturbance, the causation is reversible. Experimental sleep deprivation has been found to relieve depression or invoke a manic episode in bipolar affective disorder. On ensuring that a study sample of bipolar patients stayed awake, Thomas Wehr and fellow researchers found that even partial sleep loss was a trigger for mania.[7] The effect was temporary, patients who had been depressed slipping back after two or three days. Following an earlier observation by German psychiatrist Walter Schulte that the mood of some depressed patients improved after a sleepless night, the therapeutic possibilities of sleep deprivation has attracted research, with an active team based at the Centre of Chronobiology at the University of Basel Psychiatric Hospital. If the light of a full moon proves a sufficient stimulus for mania in bipolar disorder, perhaps the ancient idea of malevolent moonbeams was not so fanciful after all.

There is evidence that the timing of melatonin secretion varies with the mood states of manic-depressive illness.[8] Research led by Alfred Lewy of the Sleep and Mood Disorders Laboratory in Oregon has shown phase advance in mania and delay in depression. Indeed, some investigators claim that mood disorders are a result of disturbance to the body clock, a phenomenon to which Irish psychiatrist David Healy referred 'rhythm and blues'.[9] Experts such as Ellen Leibenluft have attributed rapid-cycling bipolar disorder to a dysfunctional sleep–wake cycle, with indication that decreased sleep duration precedes rather than follows a switch to mania. The endogenous type of depression shows a circadian rhythm, being most severe in the morning, and lifting in the evening. People with schizophre-

7   Wehr TA (1992): 'Improvement of depression and triggering of mania by sleep deprivation'. *Journal of the American Medical Association*, 267: 548–551.

8   Lewy AJ, Sack RL, Cutler NL, Bauer VK, Hughes RJ (1998): 'Melatonin in circadian phase sleep and mood disorders'. In *Melatonin in Psychiatric and Neoplastic Disorders* (eds M Shafii, SL Shafii). American Psychiatric Press, 81–123.

9   Healy D (1987): 'Rhythm and blues: neurochemical, neuropharmacological and neuropsychological implications of a hypothesis of a circadian rhythm dysfunction in affective disorders'. *Psychopharmacology*, 93: 271–285.

nia often turn night into day, and a longitudinal study by Russell Foster indicated that circadian regulation is poorly regulated in such patients.

Despite finding no lunar effect in their study, in 1968 psychiatrists Bauer and Hornick recommended further research on agitated patients, who could have propensity to disturbance caused by the nocturnal glow. However, little of the research on lunar influence has taken account of the brightness of night sky, which varies not only with the synodic cycle but also with meteorological conditions. One of the first studies of behaviour specifically in relation to luminosity was in 1973, but Blackman and Catalina found no statistically significant correlation with emergency room visits. Many of the studies reporting a lunar effect have found an increase in the behaviour of interest at points in the cycle other than when the Moon shines brightest; for example, Arnold Lieber reported surges in aggressive incidents at both new and full moon, thus eliminating illumination from his equation.

Nonetheless, the radiant orb continues to appeal as a cause of strange behaviour. Police in Ohio and in Kentucky have claimed that crime rises during nights with a full moon, and in 2007 Inspector Andy Parr of Sussex Police declared a plan to deploy additional officers in Brighton over summer months to counter aggressive behaviour linked to the lunar cycle. He explained: 'I compared a graph of full moons and a graph of last year's violent crimes and there is a trend. People tend to be more aggressive.'[10] This was widely reported in the British media:

Crackdown on lunar-fuelled crime (BBC website)

More police to patrol on full moons (Daily Telegraph)

Cops in full moon lunar-cy (The Sun)

Police put more officers on beat to tackle 'full-moon violence' (The Independent)

In 2008, Annette King, Justice Minister in New Zealand, suggested that a spate of stabbings could have been caused by lunar stimulation. Such anecdotal impressions should be taken with a pinch of salt. It is interesting that Inspector Parr was concerned with boisterous exploits in summertime. Thirty years ago, research by physician JP Shepherd showed that violent crime in Bristol correlated with lengthening daylight, with progressively increasing frequency of assaults from January to June. Warmer and lighter evenings tend to produce extra work for emergency services, but does the full moon have similar impact? A study in 2009 by Biermann and colleagues, using many years of records in Upper Franconia in

10   'Police put more officers on beat to tackle "full-moon violence"'. *Independent* newspaper, 6 June 2007.

Bavaria, showed no lunar periodicity with assaults, but again it should be acknowledged that research in a heterogenous population is liable to miss cyclical patterns if these occur in a minority of people.

An argument for a photic mechanism for lunacy was offered in a review in 1999 by Charles Raison, Haven Klein and Morgan Steckler at the University of California, Los Angeles. Acknowledging that lunar phases pass barely unnoticed in an urbanised society, the authors claimed that contrasts in moonlight may have had greater impact in the past, when human activity had a more natural schedule. Raison and colleagues recommended further research on psychiatric phenomena in indigenous communities in domains uncontaminated by electric lighting, where the sleep–wake cycle may continue to be influenced by changes in moonlight.

> Certain Native American people in the southwestern United States, where skies are typically clear and dark, might be ideal for such a study. Most Native Americans in this region live in isolated environments, some without electricity, others where the use of electricity is confined to indoor illumination.[11]

This historical light-contrast hypothesis has been accepted as a rational explanation by some sceptics, for whom it confines the idea of lunar influence to pre-industrial history. In their critique of lunacy research, Campbell and Beets remarked: 'Perhaps the folk beliefs concerning lunar effects were originally based on fact and only in this century have lost their validity.'[12] This suggestion was attributed by footnote to a third party (prominent behaviourist RJ Herrnstein); so sceptical were Campbell and Beets that they would not have considered this possibility themselves. Citing national statistics, Rotton and Kelly stated that as people spend most time indoors, in an artificially lit environment, behaviour is unlikely to be affected by the distant satellite. Ironically, here were the chief opponents of lunar belief accepting that the Moon can indeed affect human behaviour, but in a bygone era – not in the sunny uplands of advanced civilisation. Their rejection of lunar influence, therefore, was in the realm of applied but not pure science.

Not considered by Raison and colleagues was the environmental context of psychiatry. For most of its lifetime, the large mental institution provided unique conditions for a moonlight effect. The asylum was originally a place of refuge, intentionally isolated from the stress and vice of society. These edifices were built at elevated rural sites, designed to receive optimal sunlight and fresh air, surrounded by a vast acreage of farmland.

---

11   Raison CL, Klein HM, Steckler M (1999): 'The moon and madness reconsidered'. *Journal of Affective Disorders*, 53: 99–106.
12   Campbell and Beets (1978), p1127.

Take, for example, Netherne Hospital in Surrey, former workplace and residence of some of the nurses who inspired this book. Its red-brick maze of ward blocks and the utilities of a sizeable town encroached on the sylvan pastures of the Farthing Downs in Surrey. On the opposite side of the valley stood the monstrous former London County Council mental institution of Cane Hill; two miles north, the suburban outcrops of the metropolis; but Netherne had an air of splendid isolation. With squirrels bounding from the boughs of ornamentally-planted elms and poplars, the serenity of the grounds was incongruent with the conflict of deviance and discipline within. Yet the quality of life of residents was enriched by their pastoral surroundings, where Georgian bars framed a vista not of a smoky townscape but of green fields, and a night sky in all its glory.

On his visit to the St Vincent asylum in the Windward Islands, George Sarton attributed the alleged trouble at full moon to the outcome of staff superstition, but here was an environment free from artificial light. Some restless inmates, if not held in the deeper vaults, may have found difficulty sleeping as a brilliant moon lit their seabound sanctuary. Even in the twentieth century, away from the municipal street lighting, roads, shops and hubbub of urban ecology, the mental hospital was a relatively natural environment, thus maintaining the contrast between lunar phases. As a large proportion of admissions were of townsfolk, such monthly fluctuation from the depths of darkness to unbridled moonlight could have aggravated psychiatric symptoms. It would not be surprising if in some predisposed cases, restlessness and irritability led to manic excitement.

Unfortunately, few scientific studies of lunar influence were conducted in the former asylums. Much of the research in psychiatric services was in general hospital units or in other urban settings, where artificial lighting would have suppressed the potential impact of moonlight. In recent decades community care policy has resulted in closure of these institutions throughout the world, and so the distracting potential of a full moon noted by Haslam, Esquirol and Forbes Winslow, has been suppressed. Through technological subordination of nature, our seasonal and circadian rhythms have been blunted.[13]

---

13   Foster RG, Roenneberg T (2008): 'Human responses to the geophysical daily, annual and lunar cycles'. *Current Biology*, 18 (R): 784–794.

Seized by the Moon

A condition of special relevance to the moonlight hypothesis is epilepsy. The proportion of epileptic patients in mental hospitals remained high in the early twentieth century, when Emil Kraepelin was refining his classification of mental diseases. Initially, Kraepelin followed Pinel and other early alienists in categorising epilepsy as a neurosis, but in a later edition of his classic textbook *Psychiatrie* (1923), he placed epileptic insanity alongside dementia praecox and manic-depressive psychosis as the three most severe forms of mental illness. In a widely used manual of psychiatry in the mid-twentieth century, Henderson and Gillespie followed the psychobiological approach of Adolph Meyer in considering epilepsy as a 'reaction type'. An epileptic personality, they explained, was no longer regarded as secondary to seizures, but as a prodromal feature. The patient was typically melancholic, suspicious, self-obsessed, irritable and mentally sluggish. Illustrative case studies depicted 'turns' in behaviour, with episodes of unprovoked violence. As Henderson and Gillespie noted, the usual fate of epileptic patients was a steady decline, but a contributory factor may have been their incarceration in refractory wards. In the standard training manual for British psychiatrists from the 1950s to 1970s, Mayer-Gross, Slater and Roth stated that personality change occurred in only a minority of patients with epilepsy, but they retained the concept of epileptic dementia, and defined epileptic psychosis as a twilight state that might last many months. Debate continued about whether mental disorder was caused by chronic seizure activity, an expression of the epileptic temperament, or an iatrogenic outcome of bromide therapy.

Psychiatric interest in epilepsy *per se* waned as the concept of epileptic insanity was abandoned. Yet the epileptic population in mental hospitals remained disproportionately high, despite clinical and adminstrative developments. Whereas the asylums had historically housed patients with congenital mental defect, among whom epilepsy was common, the expansion of mental handicap institutions since the early twentieth century diverted many cases that would previously have been sent to psychiatric hospitals. There were also epileptic colonies, of which the most famous opened at Bielefeld in Germany in 1867, but such provision remained sparse. In 1946 nearly 10 per cent of the 600,000 beds for nervous or mental disease in the Unites States were occupied by epileptic patients, with the few specialist facilities housing only a quarter of these cases.[14] In 1954, at the high-water mark of the mental hospital census in England and Wales, the handful of colonies provided merely 3,622 beds for all ages.[15] A survey in 1953 by Liddell at Runwell Hospital near London showed that most epileptic patients remained in long-stay psychiatric care due to propensity to violence, troublesome personality traits and the risk of the potentially fatal crisis of status epilepticus if medication was missed.

Although mental disorder was no longer regarded as pathognomonic, epidemiological studies have shown a considerably higher frequency of psychiatric symptoms in epilepsy than in the general population. In 1966, a study of 987 epileptic patients by Gudmundsson in Iceland found that 52 per cent displayed abnormal personality features, supporting earlier observations by psychiatrists of a particular constitutional character in some cases of epilepsy. Research by TA Betts in mental hospitals in the Birmingham area revealed that a majority of chronic cases of epilepsy were initially admitted with diagnoses of furor or paranoia.[16] Betts noted their tendency to become long-stay patients; in 1965, 5 per cent of the population of psychiatric hospitals in West Midlands was epileptic.

People with epilepsy have a low seizure threshold, and are relatively sensitive to environmental disturbance such as noise or bright light. Although the Moon has long been associated with the paroxyms of epilepsy, the evidence to date is not persuasive. In 1938, on analysing records of 110 male patients, J Tylor Fox, medical superintendent of the Lingfield Epileptic Colony in Surrey, concluded that seizure patterns are endogenously regulated. Patients' activity had a weekly pattern (school for the children, domestic or farm labour for the adults, with a half-day and weekend break, church service on Sunday and midweek entertainment), but stress or excitement around the events of an otherwise monotonous routine were not reflected in seizure records. Monthly rhythms were common not only in females, in whom menstrual hormones could be blamed, but in men and boys too. However, whereas Arrhenius had found lunar periodicity in seizures, Tylor Fox found none.

Recent research has revealed some interesting temporal patterns. In a paper in 2006, Polychronopoulus and colleagues of the University of Patras Medical School in Greece reported a significant clustering of epileptic seizures at full moon at a specialist emergency clinic. Records of 859

14   Lennox WG (1946): *Science and Seizures: New Light on Epilepsy and Migraine* (2nd edition). New York: Harper & Brothers.

15   Fairfield L (1954): *Epilepsy*. London: Gerald Duckworth & Co.

16   Betts TA (1981): 'Epilepsy and the mental hospital'. In *Epilepsy and Psychiatry* (ed. EH Reynolds, MR Trimble). Edinburgh: Churchill Livingstone. 175–184.

cases admitted to the unit over a five-year period showed a startling difference: 34.2 per cent of seizures occurred in the full moon quarter, with around 22 per cent in each of the other quarters. Rüegg and colleagues (2008) found that admissions for status epilepticus to an intensive care unit peaked three days after new moon, and were lowest three days before new moon. At a Brazilian epilepsy referral centre, Terra-Bustamante and associates (2009) studied sudden unexplained deaths, an event associated with high frequency of seizures. From the records of 835 children in years 2000 to 2008, ten deaths occurred, of which seven were at full moon, although with such small numbers this finding could have been entirely due to chance.

A study by Benbadis in 2004 found no correlation with epileptic seizures, but a small but statistically significant effect was found in psychogenic non-epileptic seizures. This is a psychiatric rather than neurological phenomenon, appearing in the *DSM*. Although its defining feature is a mimic of epileptic seizures, it also occurs in a high proportion of genuine epileptic cases. Benbadis attributed the result to people with mental health problems being disproportionately influenced by astrology and other superstitions. However, the author failed to consider differences between cases of epileptic and psychogenic seizures in their use of anticonvulsant drugs. In 2008 Sallie Baxendale and Jennifer Fisher presented a sophisticated retrospective study of seizures at an epilepsy inpatient unit in London. They graded the amount of sunlit area of the Moon as a continuous quantitative variable, instead of the usual discrete moon quarters, also obtaining data on brightness of night sky from the UK Meteorology Office. The 1,571 epileptic seizures over a one-year period did not correlate with moon phases, but there were also 2,658 atypical epileptic events, and these showed a statistically significant correlation of 0.14. As found by Benbadis, this relationship occurred irrespective of the visibility of the Moon. Baxendale and Fisher attributed this to popular beliefs about full moon.

There is generally accepted evidence that seizures are related to sleep disruption, and patients with temporal lobe epilepsy are particularly susceptible.[17] Friis and Lund in 1974 showed that even people without epilepsy can suffer seizures as a result of sleep deprivation. The aforementioned study by Röösli and colleagues showing a reduction in duration of sleep at full moon has implications for an interaction between sleep, seizures and lunar cycles. In mental hospitals, an aggravating effect of moonlight on epileptic patients might explain the observation by nurses that wards were more chaotic at full moon. In 1900 Ernest White, who investi-

---

17 Rajna P, Veres J (1993): 'Correlations between night sleep duration and seizure frequency in temporal lobe epilepsy'. *Epilepsia*, 34: 574–579.

gated temporal patterns in seizures at the Dartford Asylum, suggested that the luminary stimulus might initiate a sequence of fits and aggression. One only needs to consider a packed dormitory of sixty or seventy beds to realise that a single event could easily have had a domino effect, causing a sleepless night for patients and a busy shift for nurses.

Whether or not related to the Moon, cyclical peaks and troughs in epileptic seizures would have been smoothed by the use of potent anticonvulsant medication. For many decades pharmocological treatment of epilepsy was the crude and extremely toxic bromide. Research by Langdon-Down and Brain in 1929 showed that bromide, while lessening the frequency of fits, did not affect the time distribution. From his research at the Lingfield Colony, Tylor Fox reported that phenobarbital, a slightly more effective drug, altered seizure patterns. A more effective compound was announced in 1938 by Merritt and Putman. Phenytoin had genuine antiepileptic rather than merely sedative properties. Subsequently, anticonvulsant therapy became so effective that few people with epilepsy required ongoing hospital treatment, and in many cases the destructive event of a seizure is completely preventable. The possibility of lunar influence in effectively controlled cases is therefore minimised. However, epilepsy remains an imprecisely defined condition, and it can lurk undetected for many years before diagnosis and treatment.

The aetiological relationship of epilepsy and mental disorder is complex, but in combination there may be high sensitivity to environmental stress, with moonlight just one of many possible factors contributing to mental and neurological states. As discussed in the following chapter, the Moon has other direct and indirect influences on our planet, with potentially significant impact on human behaviour.

Eight

Tidal rhythms

No man is an island entire of it self; every man is a piece of
the Continent, a part of the main.

John Donne (1624)

Traipsing along the coastal path in Cornwall at the close of a long summer
day, the author approached the cove of Portmellon with anticipation. With
coinciding full moon and perigee, a very high tide was expected around
nine o'clock in the evening, and come it did. Great waves crashed tumultu-
ously over the sea wall on to the road, dispersing flotsam and jetsam, and
plastering knots of seaweed on the window sills and roofs of the old
fishermens' cottages. From the safety of a sturdy tavern, people huddled
by the windows in awe: here was the tremendous power of the Moon on its
mother sphere, an enactment of the universal law of gravitation.

The link between ocean tides and lunar cycles was first noted by the
Greeks in the fourth century BC, but was doubted by many of the greatest
scholars of the classical era. Galileo accused Kepler of occultism for suggesting lunar regulation of the tides, the Italian attributing this to the rotation of Earth. Here was a seventeenth-century display of a conservative
tendency among scientists, whereby improbable theses are rejected outright rather than waiting for evidence. Proof finally arrived in the late seventeenth century, in Isaac Newton's *Principia*. Gravity is now known as
one of four fundamental forces in the universe, alongside electromagnetism and the strong and weak nuclear forces (a grand unified theory,
despite the efforts of Einstein and successors, remains elusive). Unlike the
polarity of electromagnetism, gravity is always positive. The lunar pull on
Earth is stronger at new and full moon, when the effect of the Moon and
Sun are combined, and maximised when either of these phases coincides
with perigee. The force is almost a third stronger when the Moon is closest
to Earth than when it is most distant.

Over the ages the morphology of the Moon has fascinated humankind,
and not only in relation to its quarterings. The moon appears dramatically

bigger and brighter when it is full and looming over the horizon, and this is not always an optical illusion; the disc is indeed 11 per cent larger from our perspective at perigee than at apogee, a visual effect enhanced when the Moon lingers at low elevation (as at harvest moon). The powers of the Moon were traditionally believed to increase with its proximity, an idea given scientific footing by the formula of Newton. Some investigators of lunar influence have focused on the apogee–perigee cycle as a causative factor. Nineteenth-century alienist Friedrich Koster observed cases of correlation between this cycle and mental symptoms, and in 1973 Klaus-Peter and Margitta Ossenkopp reported that poisoning incidents occurred more frequently around the time of perigee and apogee. However, Arnold Lieber, leading advocate of the gravitational theory of lunar influence, did not find an anomalistic effect; in his study of homicides, there was no compounding perigeal frequency on the twenty-nine occasions of coinciding full moon.

Lieber initially considered a crude mechanism for his theory of a 'biological rhythm of human aggression'.[1] Just as the ebb and flow of the oceans are governed by the Moon, the idea that bodily fluids are similarly affected has tempted many thinkers over the ages. Water is the largest constituent of all organic life on Earth, amounting to around 42 litres within the compartments of the human body. As our ratio of fluid to solids matches that of the oceans to the continents (4:1), the possibility of tidal rhythms in intercellular currents appealed to Lieber:

> My biological tides hypothesis, in its simplest form, states that the human body is susceptible to the same cosmic influences as the Earth and that the body processes ebb and flow with the tides, just as do the crust and the waters and the magnetic fields of the Earth.[2]

However, this version of microcosm/macrocosm equivalence has been debunked by scientists. Tidal forces only exist in larger volumes of water: Lake Baikal is tidal, Loch Lomond not. Landlocked stretches of water are only noticeably tidal if the area covered is wide enough for variation in gravitational pull, so that the mass of water is drawn from one side to the other by the daily motion of the Moon. Responding to Lieber's theory, astronomer George Abell explained that the impact of the Moon on bodily fluids would be extremely weak compared to that of proximate objects: one is subjected to greater gravitational force by a building across the street, or by a book held before the face.[3] Lieber speculated on 'gravoreceptors' throughout the body, possibly on neural pathways or in the walls of blood vessels, but while some organisms can apparently

1   Lieber AL, Sherin CR (1972): 'Homicides and the lunar cycle: toward a theory of lunar influence on human emotional disturbance'. *American Journal of Psychiatry*, 129: 69–74.

2   Lieber AL (1978): *The Lunar Effect*. Garden City, New York: Doubleday, p115.

3   Abell GO, Singer B (eds 1981): *Science and the Paranormal*. New York: Scribner.

detect changes in the gravitational field, there is little evidence for any influence on human behaviour. Refining his hypothesis, Lieber suggested that the synchronicity of biological rhythms with the synodic cycle is due not only to the immediate impact of gravity, but also to lunar modulation of geophysical variables, as shall now be considered.

Electromagnetic sensitivity

According to ID Kelly and K Mazurek in a critique of psychical research, 'the mind can only be directly affected by the external environment with the help of the sense organs'.[4] If referring to our quintet of vision, hearing, touch, taste and smell, this is unduly sceptical, because we could have various as yet unknown means of receiving subtle signals from the environment. Let us consider human sensitivity to electromagnetic fluctuation, a phenomenon suspected by Lieber of playing a role in his proposed behavioural rhythms. Biologists have shown that a wide range of animals navigate with the aid of magnetic information;[5] for example, migrating birds. In experiments homing pigeons have been thrown off course by the attachment of bar magnets to their necks. Neurobiologists recently identified a pair of molecules in the brain of the monarch butterfly, which spends summer in north-eastern USA or south-eastern Canada, before flying three thousand miles south to the Michoacán mountains in Mexico. The biocompass function of these molecules was confirmed when transferred to the fruit fly, which consequently displayed geomagnetic orientation. Steven Reppert at the University of Massachusetts explained that while the butterflies navigate primarily by the Sun, magnetic awareness is relied upon when the sky is cloudy.

Human beings too may be sensitive to changes in the geomagnetic field. Magnetic sensitivity was indicated in 1970 in a rigorously designed study of dowsing, the claimed ability to detect underground wells of water or oil.[6] Duane Chadwick and Larry Jensen of Utah State University found that dowsing reactions clustered around points with high magnetic field recordings. Although test bores were not dug at each selected position, the investigators attributed the participants' consistency to subterranean water causing perturbations in the geomagnetic field. There are countless

---

4   Kelly ID, Mazurek K (1983), p88.
5   Wiltschko R, Wiltschko W (2006): 'Magnetoreception'. *Bioessays*, 28: 157-168.
6   Hansen GP (1982): 'Dowsing: a review of experimental research'. *Journal of the Society for Psychical Research*, 51: 343–367.

stories of pet cats and dogs finding their way home after going astray on a family holiday, and the existence of a human compass was demonstrated in a blinded bionavigation by R Robin Baker at the University of Manchester in 1979, when high school pupils with magnets in their blindfolds showed less directional awareness than did participants wearing non-magnetic bars. As we shall see, a wide range of evidence has emerged of human electromagnetic sensitivity, although the role and mechanism are not yet understood.

In considering extrasensory mechanisms for lunar influence, Lieber referred to the novel theory presented forty years earlier by Harold Saxton Burr. Professor of anatomy at Yale, Burr spent most of his career developing his theory of life fields, positing the entire organisation of the universe as an electrodynamic system governing organic life through control of the movement and position of all charged particles. 'L-fields', he claimed, exist in each living organism as previously undetected bands of the electromagnetic spectrum, maintaining harmony in the disparate tissues and bodily processes. Working with colleague FSC Northrop at their laboratory at New Haven in Connecticut, Burr used voltometers to measure electrical potential in trees, rabbits, parakeets and human beings, presenting initial findings in the treatise *The Electro-Dynamic Theory of Life* in 1935. His primitive meters would have generated more noise than signal, but were sufficiently sensitive to differentiate between positive and negative polarity. L-field activity suggested a regulatory function in certain biological processes such as tumours, healing, drug effects and sleep. Accumulating data over several decades, Burr found that electrical readings in trees correlated with sunspot cycles, thunderstorms and phases of the Moon.

Results from human subjects led Burr to claim an intimate link between cosmic events and health. The medical potential of L-field theory was demonstrated when cancerous activity in the female genito-urinary tract was predicted by electrical recordings, before any clinical signs had appeared. However, Burr's research was not published in leading journals, but mostly in the *Yale Journal of Biology and Medicine*, which he edited. Burr made increasingly extravagant claims in later years, and his potentially important findings received little attention from biologists, or from mainstream medicine, where the concept of an invisible force was likely to evoke connotations with the discredited vitalism and animal magnetism of the past.

After a chance meeting with Burr at a summer party in 1947, Yale neuropsychiatrist Leonard J Ravitz was inspired into pursuing electrodynamic theory in his specialty. Borrowing a voltometer from Burr, Ravitz began by recording baseline L-fields in mentally stable people, producing norms for reference in psychiatric assessment. Detection of the very weak signal being prone to instrument bias, Ravitz made painstaking efforts to refine his toolkit of millivoltmeters and electrodes; an impedance range of 10 to 1,000 megohms was deemed satisfactory to minimise current flow from subject to device. From 1950 onwards he performed longitudinal measurement of patients with schizophrenia and manic-depressive illness at the School of Medicine at Duke University, North Carolina. A return to normal electrical state appeared to predict recovery, indicating that a patient may be ready for discharge; spikes in voltage gradient suggested imminent relapse. He analogised schizophrenia, with its alternating states of excitation and withdrawal, to an overcharged car battery, which cannot hold a charge for long and eventually burns out. An extreme electrical swing was observed in a patient shifting from schizophrenic torpor to animated volition. In controlled experiments he measured electrical activity in various depths of hypnosis, finding peak readings during emotional discharge. Ravitz explained: 'Emotional activity and stimuli of any sort involve mobilization of electrical energy, as indicated on the galvanometer; hence, both emotions and stimuli evoke the same energy. Emotions can be equated with energy.'[7]

Ravitz asserted that periodicities in medical conditions should be understood as 'electrocyclic phenomena'. In a 57-page paper in the *Annals of the New York Academy of Science* in 1962, he described a series of case studies, including twin brothers with schizophrenia, in which psychotic or affective symptoms increased at full or new moon. Convinced of a direct influence of the electromagnetic environment on mental and physical health from over fifty years of research, in 2002 Ravitz crystallised his findings in the book *Electrodynamic Man*. While most psychiatrists may be unaware of this work, the therapeutic importance of electromagnetism is becoming more apparent to the discipline, with growing interest in mild brain stimulation (as discussed later in this chapter).

Medical application of electromagnetism became widespread in the nineteenth century following the discovery of alternating current by Michael Faraday, with enthusiasts including several asylum doctors, but in 1910 the Flexner Report for the American Medical Association found no scientific basis for such treatments, leading to the demise of this trial-and-error adventure. After a long hibernation, electrical medicine was revived in the 1960s, with an outstanding figure in orthopaedic surgeon Robert O Becker (1924–2008) at the State University of New York. Intrigued by Burr's report of subtle differences in electrical potential between healthy and injured tissue, Becker pursued the clinical implications in limb repair. Performing experimental amputations on salamanders, an amphibian with high regenerative response to injury, Becker

---

7   Ravitz LJ (1962): 'History, measurement, and applicability of periodic changes in the electromagnetic field in health and disease'. *Annals of the New York Academy of Science*, 98: 1144–1201.

discovered a sequence of electrical changes at the stump. Observing that nerve tissue produces a miniscule amount of direct-current electricity at a wound site, he hypothesised an additional means of communication in the nervous system (independent of the known transmission route via the synapse between neurones), which controls slower processes of growth and healing. This direct-current circuit, according to Becker, is conducted by the glial cells. Although they outnumber neurones, these cells were regarded by anatomists as merely the glue of the nervous system, and it was not believed that they relayed messages. Becker challenged this view, finding that the membranes of glial cells held fluctuating electrical charge, which is necessarily influenced by external electromagnetic energy.

Following the success in 1967 of Stephen D Smith of University of Kentucky in promoting growth through implanting batteries in the leg stumps of frogs, Becker proved the principle of electrically-induced regeneration in mammals by achieving substantial limb repair in rats. In the 1970s he began electrical treatment in patients, initially as a last resort for complicated cases. Becker found that by applying a silver electrode to the affected part, he could resolve the two major problems of orthopaedics: osteomyelitis and non-union. First, application of positive electrical charge killed the bacteria of bone infection without damaging healthy tissue; second, reluctant union could be encouraged with negative charge. With obvious carcinogenic hazards in inducing cell differentiation, and inevitable associations with Doctor Frankenstein in the popular media, Becker warned against cavalier experimentalism. While the potential of electromagnetic therapy is yet to be fully realised, advanced technology has been developed to augment the healing process in bone, tendons and cartilage, nerves and spinal cord, and patented devices are available for pain management in childbirth. The momentum is maintained by international bodies such as the Bioelectromagnetic Society, and various peer-reviewed journals.

In his later career, Becker claimed to have found the missing link between bioenergetic and geomagnetic cycles.[8] On a government commission to investigate acupuncture, he observed elevated electrical signal at the treatment points on the classical meridian lines. Although no anatomical features are consistent with this model, Becker's finding suggested that the acupuncture points act as conductors of a direct current, which is manipulated by the treatment. He concluded that the magnetic field generated by his speculated perineural growth and repair control system involves the same low-frequency electromagnetic field exploited for two

8   Becker RO (1972): 'Electromagnetic forces and life processes'. *Technology Review*, 75: 2–8.

thousand years by Oriental medicine.[9] Electromagnetism, according to Becker, is not only the *modus operandi* of *qi gong* and other eastern faith healing, but also for extrasensory perception and other paranormal activity. The location of electromagnetic detection is not known, but Becker described the multifunctional pineal gland as our 'third eye'.

Becker then got himself embroiled in controversy. Appointed to a committee on a proposed submarine communication system in Wisconsin, he presented findings from bioelectromagnetic research in the Soviet Union indicating potential harm to human population. He also got involved in campaigns against planned power lines, but his warnings were challenged by scientists hired by energy companies, and cost him badly in further research funding. However, there are persisting health concerns about the invisible dangers of electropollution. Of growing relevance today is Becker's prophecy that electronic communication systems would cause an epidemic of neuroplastic disease due to excessive exposure to electromagnetic waves, and that governments and industry would conspire with their chosen experts to dismiss health concerns. Parts of his *magnum opus* of 1985, *Body Electric: Electromagnetism and the Foundation of Life*, read like a late twentieth-century version of the 'railway sickness' scare, with prophecies of doom, of birth defects and cancer resulting from use of office computers, but he raised pertinent concerns about the longer-term effects of electromagnetic appliances.[10] Leukaemia is a condition repeatedly but inconclusively linked to extremely low-frequency electromagnetic fields, and there may be serious mental health effects. 1979 Becker collaborated with British physician F Stephen Perry, who had noticed in his practice in Wolverhampton a disproportionate frequency of depression among patients living near overhead power lines, and their research showed an increased incidence of suicide.

With the immense growth in communication technology, human beings have dramatically altered the natural electromagnetic environment, but our activities are trivial compared to the powers of the Sun. The eleven-year sunspot cycle was first described in 1843 by amateur German astronomer Heinrich Samuel Schwabe, but sunspots were not understood until 1908, when American astronomer George Ellery Hale, using a spectroheliograph, concluded that the dark patches were indicative of

---

9   Exponents may argue that *qi* is a fundamentally deeper source of energy, beyond the explanatory grasp of western physics. However, it is interesting that most acupuncturists now use electrical apparatus rather than needles, which avoids discomfort, and apparently produces more lasting results.

10   Recently the International Union of Radio Science launched a commission to investigate the impact of electromagnetism on biology and medicine. We must hope that investigators will be allowed to disseminate politically unfavourable findings without constraint.

intense magnetic fields.[11] The connection was thus made between sunspots and magnetic storms. When sunspots appear, large amounts of ionised particles and electrons are thrown from the Sun. A solar flare is witnessed nine minutes after it occurs (according to the speed of light), but projected particles take three days to reach Earth. These missiles would be highly destructive were it not for their deflection by our invisible geomagnetic shield, but some highly charged particles permeate the atmosphere at the poles, creating the phenomenon of the Northern Lights and its southern hemisphere equivalent. Solar storms interfere with the geomagnetic field lines, sometimes shifting the position of our magnetic poles, causing considerable inaccuracies in navigation equipment. Signal from television and mobile telephone satellites can be severely disrupted, and a few years ago a surge in sunspot activity caused a short circuit in the Canadian power grid. Various organic processes have been found to reflect the sunspot cycle; for example, the girth of rings in tree trunks.

During magnetic storms, the strength of the magnetic field around Earth can fluctuate by as much as 10 per cent. Geomagnetic influences on mental health were first reported in a German medical journal in 1935, by T Düll and B Düll. Analysis of 40,000 cases over a period of five years revealed correlation between magnetic storms and incidence of neurological and psychological disturbance, including suicides. Robert Becker collaborated with psychiatrist Howard Friedman in the 1960s to study magnetic influences on mental health; from data on 28,000 admissions to eight New York psychiatric hospitals, they found increases around the time of magnetic storms, of which sixty-seven occurred during the 4-year period. In 1994 psychiatrist Ronald Kay also found correlation with magnetic storms, using admissions data from the Lothian Psychiatric Case Register, although statistical significance was limited to psychotic depression in males. Israeli researchers reported an increase in psychiatric admissions during periods of positive ionisation in the geomagnetosphere.[12] In healthy subjects researchers have observed disorganised functional activity in the brain during geomagnetic disturbances, manifesting in headaches and lethargy.

In his eloquent narrative on the Sun, Richard Cohen hinted that it was perhaps not by chance alone that the French, American and both Russian revolutions coincided with solar eruptions.[13] Perhaps historians might

11 Hale (1868–1938) spent long periods in sanatoria for recurring nervous and mental afflictions, including frequent headaches and schizophrenia, and he claimed that an elf visited him regularly to advise on his work.

12 Raps A , Soupel E, Shimshoni M (1991): 'Solar activity and admissions of psychiatric inpatients, relations and possible implications on seasonality'. *Israeli Journal of Psychiatry and Related Sciences*, 28: 72–80.

13 Cohen R (2010): *Chasing the Sun: The Epic Story of the Star that Gives Us Life*. London: Simon & Schuster.

also consider the timing of tumultuous events in relation to the Moon. Since the 1960s evidence has confirmed that our satellite exerts a tidal influence on the geomagnetic field, with activity increasing by around 4 per cent in the days following full moon.[14] In 1966 B Bell and R Defouw observed that the force is strongest when full and new moons occur closest to the ecliptic. As the geomagnetic shield is influenced by the Moon, lunar cycles affect the deflection and entry of charged particles emanating from sunspots. Becker argued that his direct current control system, being tuned into the electromagnetic field of Earth, would necessarily be influenced by solar and lunar cycles.

A possible mechanism for lunar influence, as discussed by Salvatore Garzino in his review, is through response of serotonin levels in the brain to atmospheric ion concentration, causing irritability and depression. Discovered by biologist Betty Twarog in 1952, serotonin plays a major role in psychiatric aetiology. Excess or deficit in its throughput at the synapse between neurones is the target of psychopharmacology, particulary antidepressants. Responding to the lunar-serotonin conjecture, critic David Campbell emphasised that as ion fluctuations mostly relate to climate and pollution on Earth itself, the Moon would have trivial impact. Fellow sceptics Rotton and Kelly had 'the impression that investigators are invoking one set of mysteries to explain another'.[15] Nonetheless, with evidence of a small but statistically significant correlation between geomagnetism and mental disturbance, and monthly perturbations in magnetic activity caused by the Moon, an indirect lunar influence on behaviour via geophysical forces is in principle a reasonable hypothesis.

Lunar influence on weather

For millennia farmers have predicted weather by the Moon, and the first scientific evidence of a relationship was provided by meteorologist Giuseppe Toaldo (1719–1797). Analysing records in Padova, he attributed monthly patterns to reflection of solar heat by the Moon. Another potential meteorological influence was through atmospheric tides, which were first described in 1746 by French astronomer–mathematician Jean d'Alembert (1717–1783), and studied by Laplace and Lamarck in the late eighteenth century. Like oceanic tides, atmospheric tides have daily and monthly

---

14 As reported by Stolov HL, Cameron AGW (1964): 'Variations of geomagnetic activity with lunar phase'. *Journal of Geophysical Research*, 69: 4975–4982.
15 Rotton and Kelly (1985a), p289.

rhythms, regulated by the orbital position of the Moon. However, barometric measurement showed only a weak effect of these tides. Unlike water, air has little mass upon which lunar gravitation can draw. In the early nineteenth century, astronomers Wilhelm Olbers and Johann Heinrich Mädler concluded that the Moon was unlikely to have any significant effect on the weather, whether through heat, light, gravity or any other means. More recently, analysis of daily temperature records from 1979 to 1994 by Balling and Cerveny showed a thermal variation between new and full moon of merely 0.02°C.

There is stronger evidence of a lunar effect on rain. In 1962 two papers in *Science* journal confirmed the discovery of over a hundred years earlier by Italian astronomer Giovanni Schiaparelli (1835–1910) that precipitation and cloud cover correlate with phases of the Moon. DA Bradley, MA Woodbury and GW Brier analysed data from 1,544 North American weather stations from 1900 to 1949, finding disproportionately higher frequency of heavy rain just after new and full moon. EE Adderley and EG Bowen found similar association in twenty-five years of records from fifty weather stations in New Zealand. Acknowledging lunar periodicity in hurricanes and tropical storms, climatologists believe that the Moon modulates precipitation by displacing anticyclones.

The weather has long been associated with mental disorder, particularly in relation to temperature and humidity. Among early alienists, Pinel and Guislain noted that attacks in periodical insanity increased after spring solstice and fell in autumn; Reil mentioned approaching thunderstorms as a trigger. Research has confirmed seasonal variations, with a disproportionate incidence of suicide in spring,[16] and of mania in summer.[17] Evidence of a relationship between barometric pressure and mental disturbance appeared in the *American Journal of Psychiatry* in the 1930s: Mills reported an increase in suicides at times of low pressure and heat, and Hoverson found a tendency for acute psychotic reactions to follow electrical storms. Geographically specific winds are an alleged cause of restlessness and agitation. The *föhn* of the Swiss mountains is a dry wind blowing down the leeward slopes, which can raise temperatures by as much as 30°C in a few hours, dramatically clearing deep layers of snow. Austrian physician Anton Czermak first described its health effects in the nineteenth century, and while studies have shown increases in suicide and accidents, *föhnkrankheit* is a phenomenon yet to be fully investigated.

Some investigators of lunar influence on behaviour have considered indirect causation through meteorological patterns. From 1920 to 1950,

---

16   Swinscow D (1951): 'Some suicide statistics'. *British Medical Journal*, i: 1417-1423.
17   Symonds RL, Williams P (1976): 'Seasonal variations in the incidence of mania'. *British Journal of Psychiatry*, 129: 45–48.

William F Peterson conducted biometeorological research at the University of Illinois Medical School in Chicago. He reported correlations of weather patterns with births, deaths, epileptic seizures and suicides, with intervening effects of solar and lunar cycles. Interpreting their observed rise in self-poisoning incidents at apogee and perigee, Klaus Peter and Margitta Ossenkopp speculated an indirect effect of the Moon on weather formations, through its interference with the geomagnetic field. Sheldon Geller and Herbert Shannon in 1976 reported that psychiatric contacts at a Toronto hospital increased with an interaction between full moon and high humidity. Other studies have found no compounding effect of lunar cycles and weather on mental symptoms.

The few positive findings may have been due to confounding variables such as solar activity. Meteorologist Damio Camuffo at the Institute of Atmospheric Science and Climate in Italy argues that forecasting weather by the Moon would be to dabble in the merest of probabilities, lunar position being one of multiple factors in a complex and chaotic system. As in the popular illustration of chaos theory (the mathematics of non-linear dynamic systems), a single flap of a butterfly's wings in Patagonia can set off a chain of events culminating in thunderstorms on the other side of the world. A fundamental goal of science is prediction, but determining future lunar effects would be unfeasibly difficult. Of course, the same could be said of long-term weather outlooks generally. The Met Office in Britain has a tarnished record of late, its elaborate computer models promising a 'barbecue summer' in 2009, which transpired as the coolest for decades. The weather would be an unreliable medium for lunacy.

It is not disputed that the Moon affects atmospheric tides and the weather, but physician Daniel Myers concluded that the impact can be quantified as 'physiologically insignificant'.[18] Myers supported his argument with a battery of facts and figures: atmospheric tides are more of a thermal than a gravitational phenomenon; lunar contribution to barometric pressure is slight (of a maximum magnitude of 0.02mmHg, while normal barometric pressure at sea level is 760mmHg); of tidal fluctuations in the geomagnetic field, 95 per cent is caused by the Sun, leaving only 5 per cent to the Moon. On existing scientific evidence, a lunar link may seem tortuous, but it is theoretically possible that the modest effect of lunar cycles on air flow and the geomagnetosphere could be reflected in people vulnerable to mental imbalance. We shall now focus on a psychiatric condition in which environmental stress is particularly relevant.

18   Myers DE (1995): 'Gravitational effects of the period of high tides and the new moon on lunacy'. *Journal of Emergency Medicine*, 13: 529–532.

Ebb and flow in mood disorder

Before manic-depressive psychosis was established by Kraepelin as a specific psychiatric condition, alienists saw mania and melancholia in the same patient as a comorbidity, but the idea of a combined syndrome has older origins. As George Man Burrows described in his *Commentaries on Insanity* of 1828, Roman physicians understood the two affective extremes as an interchangeable disorder of passions, and Thomas Willis analogised melancholia and mania as smoke and flame. However, as historian of psychiatry German Berrios has explained, mania had a quite different meaning in the past than in modern psychiatry. In the nineteenth century, mania was the most common diagnosis in asylums. The label did not only mean an affective state of extreme elation but covered all kinds of delusional ideation and irrational behaviour; indeed, it was often used as a generic term for insanity. Many of the cases of mania diagnosed by alienists would today be labelled as schizophrenic.

Identification of mania and depression as a single category of mental disorder is credited to two alienists at the Salpêtrière in Paris: Jean-Pierre Falret, head of the institution since 1831; and Jules Baillarger, who had founded *Annales Médico-Psychologiques*, the leading French psychiatric journal. In his lectures at the Salpêtrière and in contributions to the *Gazette des Hôpitaux* in 1851, Falret presented a rotational syndrome of mania and melancholia. He did not name this condition until three years later, after Baillarger had identified *folie à double forme,* which featured a swing from mania to depression followed by remission, in a single or repeated sequence. Falret described an enduring illness, with a perpetual cycle of mania, depression and lucid intervals. A bitter dispute ensued over priority, but it was Falret who most closely described the condition later established as a major disease category of modern psychiatry. From longitudinal case studies, Karl Kahlbaum (1828–1899) classified two types of cyclical insanity: *Vecordie* and *Vesania tipica*. While the former had benign outcome, the latter led to dementia, thus sowing the seeds for his fellow Prussian in differentiating manic-depressive psychosis and dementia praecox. In a paper of 1882 Kahlbaum introduced the term 'cyclothymia' for a mild form of the disorder, which rarely required asylum treatment. He suggested that this previously unknown condition was highly prevalent in society, sufferers complaining when depressed without noticing a contrasting period of elevated mood ('hyperthymia') as an abnormality.

Kraepelin introduced manic-depressive disorder in the sixth edition of his textbook in 1899. As many symptoms were shared with dementia praecox, the fundamental difference was intervening lucidity. Various fluctuating and temporary states were brought into the manic-depressive category, but Kraepelin's formulation was not immediately accepted beyond central Europe, partly due to anti-German sentiment following the Great War, and a time lag in translation for the English-speaking world. As David Healy told in his history of mania, the French continued to refer to *la folie circulaire*, while in Britain and America, chronic states of affective extremes were diagnosed sooner or later as dementia praecox. The manic-depressive disease category was propagated by psychiatrists migrating *en masse* from Nazi Germany, but diagnosis was relatively rare until the widespread availability of pharmaceutical treatment in the 1960s. Dissatisfaction with pessimistic aspects of Kraepelin's manic-depressive psychosis eventually led to its reformulation as bipolar mood disorder, which appeared in the third edition of the *DSM-III* classification system in 1980.

A common presentation of bipolar affective disorder is a cyclical pattern of mood swings. Writing in 1913, Kraepelin did not regard cyclicity as a distinguishing feature of manic-depressive psychosis because it also appeared in epileptic and hysterical illness; also, manic and depressive phases did not necessarily follow a regular sequence. However, seasonal patterns occur in manic and depressive episodes, and some patients show remarkably consistent rotation from pole to pole, often with monthly or six-weekly cycles. Cases in the lunar research of Friedrich Koster would almost certainly be diagnosed with bipolar affective disorder today. In his research at Birmingham mental hospitals in the 1950s, John Crammer found patients with manic-depressive disorder or catatonic schizophrenia with recurring sequences of brief admissions to hospital, spontaneous recovery, a period of stability, relapse at home and readmission. Further examples were found on the 'back wards', where ward staff could confidently predict that a patient was 'due a turn', although such periodicity was rarely reflected in medical notes. Crammer noted that once patterns were established, they tended to persist.

Fortnightly and monthly periodicity featured prominently in the works of Hippocrates and Galen, but generalised temporal regulation was discarded in post-humoural medicine, except in infectious diseases. In the late nineteenth century Wilhem Fliess (1858–1928) of Berlin was studying patterns of fever outbreaks when he heard of an intriguing cyclicity in dreams and in infant behaviour described by psychologist Herman Svoboda in Vienna. Fliess attempted to confirm these putative rhythms of twenty-three days in physical health and twenty-eight days in the nervous system, the latter manifesting in changes in mood and sensitivity. To the physical and emotional patterns was added an intellectual cycle in the 1920s by Alfred Teltscher, who observed a thirty-three-day rhythm in performance of engineering students at the University of Innsbruck; in the first sixteen days of their individual periods, students were more able to absorb and apply complex information.

Indexed on date of birth, the trinity of cycles became known as biorhythms. Vitality peaks in the ascendant phase of each cycle, declining in the descendant or recuperative phase. A minor industry emerged in the production of personal charts, but despite mass popularity in the mid-twentieth century, biorhythms have never been supported by medical research. In 1981 Winstead, Schwartz and Bertrand found no evidence of biorhythms in psychiatric admissions in New Orleans. However, the authors acknowledged that by including all diagnostic categories, they would have missed any specific effects in cyclical conditions, as in the mood swings of manic-depressive illness. Indeed, bipolar affective disorder often shows patterns similar to that described by Fliess. The pseudoscience of biorhythms fell from fashion, but some basis may yet be found in physiological and behavioural cycles through the proper scientific discipline of chronobiology. Although the emotional cycle in biorhythms was of similar duration to the lunar cycle, natal determination left no room for environmental factors, whereas chronobiologists consider physiological rhythms as intrinsically regulated systems of potential extrinsic synchronisation. The contrast mirrors that between astrology and astronomy.

Cyclical patterns in bipolar disorder could be caused by disturbance of normal endogenous rhythms, possibly as an excessive response to environmental stimuli. On discussing observed fluctuation in psychiatric symptoms, Crammer hypothesised a fault in homeostasis, a term coined by American neurologist Walter Bradford Cannon (1871–1945) for the concept of regulatory feedback systems to maintain constancy in the body. Crammer suggested that patients are prone to attacks at particular points of a biochemical rhythm, when stress might instigate an ordered sequence of symptoms. A possible cue is menstruation, which commonly featured in the aetiological observations of nineteenth-century alienists. Indeed, there are gender differences in bipolar affective disorder, Ellen Leibenluft in 1996 observing that rapid cycling occurs more frequently in females, probably due to hormonal rhythms. In women with periods of circalunar duration, the irritability, anxiety and mood swings often occurring in premenstrual tension would produce at least a coincidental lunar pattern. If both lunar phase entrainment and an aggravating menstrual effect in bipolar disorder were confirmed, there could be sufficient causal evidence to vindicate ancient links between Moon, mind and menses. Female lunar periodicity was described in the eighteenth-century cases of Richard Mead:

> The girl, who was of lusty full habit of body, continued well for a few days, but was at full moon again seized with a most violent fit, after which, the disease kept its periods constant and regular with the tides; she lay always speechless during the whole time of flood, and recovered upon the ebb.[19]

Reports of correlating affective, menstrual and lunar cycles remain at anecdotal level, with so many confounding factors that a link with the Moon may seem tortuous. Ravitz described such temporal patterns in manic-depressive patients, his charts showing voltage extremes at new and full moon, as in this 42-year-old woman:

> Her greatest perturbations tended to approximate lunar syzygies. Premenstrual tension symptoms began one day before new moon, on May 22, and extended into her period, ending on June 1, an interval of considerable voltage flux. None preceded her menstrual period on June 20 to 22, during a period of low field intensity and minimal variability. Following the menstrual period, depressive-tension symptoms began to develop, reaching their maximum on June 25, three days after new moon, associated with pronounced field intensification in the plus direction. The tension component then dropped out, with augmentation of the depressive features. During the following negative excursion, she was felt to be suicidal, on June 27. A short-lived depresive- tension state preceded the July menstrual period during intensifications in the minus direction.[20]

Bipolar affective disorder was considered in a recent paper by Koukopoulus as a problem of energy depletion. Manic attacks exhaust the body, counteracting the biological processes that supply energy, and a subsequent depressive episode may be an enforced means of recuperation. The primacy of mania in the cycle is supported by the fact that treatments for bipolar disorder are basically antimanic agents; by thwarting mania, they also prevent the rebound depresssion. Furthermore, patients whose cycles begin with manic episodes are known to respond better to prophylactic drugs.[21] Treatment for manic-depressive disorder originated in a serendipitous observation in 1949 by Australian psychiatrist John Cade. Lithium salts were being used to reduce uric acid in the blood, and as it induced drowsiness Cade hypothesised that mania was caused by excessive urea. He tested this substance on a group of manic patients and found that their excitation was interrupted, only to resume once lithium

19   Mead R (1746): 'Treatise concerning the influence of the Sun and Moon upon human bodies, and the diseases thereby produced'. In *The Medical Works of Richard Mead*. Dublin: Thomas Ewing, pp113–156.

20   Ravitz (1962), pp1168–1170.

21   Koukopoulus A, Sani G, Koukopoulus AE, Albert MJ, Girardi P, Taterelli R (2006): 'Endogenous and exogenous cyclicity and temperament in bipolar disorder: review, new data and hypotheses'. *Journal of Affective Disorders*, 96: 165–175.

was withdrawn. Diagnoses of manic-depressive disorder increased in the 1970s once cost-benefit analysis had confirmed the merits of lithium as effective prophylaxis. Initially tardy drug company interest was probably due to the substance being naturally occurring (number three in the periodic table of elements), precluding its potential as a patented product.

Patients with cyclical mood swings would appear to offer an untapped potential for research on lunar influence. However, use of mood stabilising medication is an obstacle in studying naturalistic patterns in patients with bipolar affective disorder. Although it would be fascinating to isolate groups of people with specific psychiatric conditions on a remote hillside free from artificial light and neuroleptic drugs, to deprive patients of proven treatment for a study of apparently limited clinical value would not be looked upon favourably by a research ethics committee. Nonetheless, the pharmacological blanket may be permeable. Lieber noted that manic-depressive patients would often contact him around the same time, troubled by restlessness and insomnia. Blood tests showed that their lithium levels had dipped below the therapeutic range, and a temporary dose increase was necessary to suppress the symptoms. Rather more persuasive evidence of lunar periodicity would be needed for such treatment adjustment to become standard practice.

Borderlands of mania and epilepsy

Originating in the Hippocratic corpus, a putative affinity between mood disorders and epilepsy continues to draw interest from neurologists and neuropsychiatrists, with observed similarities in course, symptoms and cyclicity. Mood disturbances are common in epilepsy, while many patients with bipolar affective disorders have epileptoid features. The boundaries between psychiatric and neurological symptology are never static, and the possibility of an interactive complex would involve the two conditions traditionally associated with the Moon.

In the early asylum era, when epilepsy was rampant among inmates, alienists regarded seizures as a manifestation of mental disorder. In the mid-nineteenth century Krafft-Ebing likened a state occurring before mania to a pre-epileptic aura, manifested by heart palpitations and neuralgic signs, with behavioural disturbances such as irritability, destructive activity and sexual promiscuity. Several writers reckoned that maniacal outbursts sometimes replaced seizures. Before Kraepelin had added epileptic insanity to complete his trinity of severe mental disorders,

Ziehen in 1902 described composite psychoses, which he divided into periodic and non-periodic types;[22] Henrichsen in 1911 suggested that some manic-depressive states were actually a presentation of epilepsy rather than true manic-depressive disease; Ritterhaus in 1920 surmised a common aetiology, having observed epileptic manifestations in manic-depressive psychosis including spasms, twilight states, confusional delirium and personality features. Others such as Krisch in 1922 believed that while the conditions sometimes coexisted with overlapping features, they remained independent. In their textbook of the 1950s, Mayer-Gross, Slater and Roth saw no difficulty in differentiating the affective symptoms of epileptic periodicity and manic-depressive psychosis, but they hinted at a hereditary comorbidity.

Better understanding of the sequential relationship between epilepsy and mental disorder requires a closer relationship between psychiatry and neurology, branches of medicine that have developed in Cartesian parallel. Psychiatry has generally shown limited interest in *rapprochement* with neurology, perhaps fearing imposition of naïve physical science on the maze of mental disorder, and a possible loss of status were *psyche* to be overshadowed by *soma* in aetiology, assessment and treatment. However, since the 1960s, some biologically orientated psychiatrists, encouraged by neurological discoveries in mental disorders, have attempted to build collaboration beyond a few conditions in 'no man's land'. As all mental symptoms have associated biological action (whatever the direction of relationship), much may be gained from a coalescence of neurological and psychiatric expertise.

A therapeutic window had been opened in Budapest in 1934, when Ladislaus von Meduna launched his convulsive treatment for schizophrenia, initially through injection of camphor oil. Paracelsus had used camphor in the sixteenth century as an assault on severe mental disturbance, and there are occasional mentions of analeptic treatment from the pre-psychiatry era, but Meduna was first to present a rational thesis for the therapeutic application of seizures. Finding camphor unreliable, Meduna switched to Cardiazol, a synthetic camphor solution used as a cardiac stimulant. Although he considered epilepsy and schizophrenia as opposite poles of a psychoneurological continuum, Meduna's theoretical basis has been misrepresented. He was well aware that psychosis and epilepsy sometimes appeared in the same patient. At the same institution in Budapest, Nyïro and Jablonszky had identified schizophrenic traits in 81 of 176 epileptic patients, and Meduna saw therapeutic implications in the observation that cases with psychotic features tended to have a favourable

---

22   For a detailed account see Berrios GE (1979): 'Insanity and epilepsy in the nineteenth century'. In *Psychiatry, Genetics and Pathography: a Tribute to Eliot Slater* (eds M Roth, V Cowie). London: Gaskell.

prognosis. In a historical review, Wolf and Trimble suggested that Meduna actually meant symptomatic antagonism within syndromic affinity; in other words, opposite sides of the same coin.[23]

The biochemical mechanism of convulsive therapy was pursued in earnest by a profession heartened by this therapeutic revolution. Advances in neurological investigation raised prospects of revealing not only the biological action of Cardiazol and its replacement ECT, but more importantly the pathological process of schizophrenia. Electrical activity in the brain had been measurable since 1929, when German psychiatrist Hans Berger introduced the electro-encephalograph. This instrument amplified and graphically displayed the rhythmic pulsations of neurones, with normal 'brain waves' escalating to a 'brain storm' during an epileptic seizure. The EEG became an important diagnostic tool, but there was no straightforward diagnosis from electrical recordings. Harvard neurologists FA Gibbs, EL Gibbs and WG Lennox found that abnormalities typical of epilepsy occurred in as many as 10 per cent of the general population, most of whom lacked any epileptic tendencies. In 1938 they reported that epileptoid waves were particularly common in schizophrenic patients.

The relationship between epilepsy and schizophrenia faded from psychiatric interest in the 1940s, but the idea was kept alive by a few neurologically-orientated practitioners. On finding that subcortical discharges correlated with the recovery process in schizophrenics, Denis Hill in 1950 proposed a homeostatic theory whereby psychosis is corrected by seizures, and *vice versa*. In 1953 Hans Landolt discovered that behavioural disturbance in epileptics during seizure-free periods brought a return to normal EEG readings, a phenomenon he called 'forced normalisation'. Since then several writers have considered the mutually protective effect of seizures and schizophrenic episodes, Stevens describing a *yin* and *yang* relationship, with each condition a polarised response to imbalance in excitatory and inhibitory networks.[24] Such theories are contested, an antagonistic phenomenon being demonstrated in only a few cases.

Again, a confounding factor is the use of maintenance medication, but such treatment may also provide clues to explaining the epileptic-psychotic relationship. Strong tranquillisers sometimes provoke seizures, while highly retardant anticonvulsants such as phenobarbitone and phenytoin are psychotogenic. Pharmacologocal intervention, while controlling *grand mal* seizures, may generate complex partial seizures with mental effects. An antagonistic mechanism could be activated or sup-

23 Wolf P, Trimble MR (1985): 'Biological antagonism and epileptic psychosis'. *British Journal of Psychiatry*, 146: 272–276.

24 Stevens JR (1998): 'Seizure or psychosis: alternative brain responses to the physiological events of puberty, the reproductive period, brain injury or malformation'. In *Forced Normalization and Alternative Psychoses of Epilepsy* (eds Trimble MR, Schmitz B). Petersfield: Wrightson Biomedical. 121–141.

pressed by medicinal or shock treatments. Although it transpired that the true therapeutic indication for convulsive therapy is depressive illness, schizophrenia of catatonic type or with a prominent affective component also appeared to respond. Meduna accepted the limitations of Cardiazol in reversing chronic schizophrenia, but claimed that patients requiring lower doses for seizure were amenable to complete recovery. Convulsive therapy possibly stimulated an antagonistic mechanism in an as yet unidentified psychotic syndrome. EEG investigations showed that whereas the spontaneous seizures of idiopathic epilepsy tend to develop in foci and spread by conduction, Cardiazol had a sudden widespread impact on the brain. Repeated applications of convulsive therapy, while producing transient improvement, possibly blunt an innate inhibitory response.

Such a protective mechanism is possibly impaired as schizophrenia progresses. Of relevance here is the other 'shock treatment' of the 1930s. Insulin coma therapy, introduced by Manfred Sakel in Vienna, was a dangerous and labour intensive treatment, but was believed to act at a deeper level in delusional psychoses (little love was lost between Meduna and Sakel, who both claimed primacy in physical treatment of schizophrenia). Observing patients at the insulin coma department at Bethlem Royal Hospital, Hoenig and Leibermann reported in 1953 that seizure threshold fluctuated with schizophrenic states, being highest in stupor, and lowest at point of recovery.[25] While convulsive therapy induces a generalised tonic-clonic *grand mal* seizure, insulin coma placed patients in a prolonged epileptogenic situation. Although seizures and spasms were regarded by Sakel and most practitioners as an adverse event, their therapeutic value may have been underestimated. Insulin coma therapy was abandoned in the late 1950s in favour of the convenient and less hazardous neuroleptic drugs, and the potential convulsive link was missed.

While ECT is not recommended for chronic conditions due to the neurological sequelae of multiple courses, an analeptic agent of lesser potency is currently being tested. First used by neurologists in the 1980s as a diagnostic tool, transcranial magnetic stimulation (TMS) has mood-enhancing effects, and can provoke seizures in patients with a low threshold. In 1995, testing TMS in depression, Kolbinger and colleagues found best results in a group of patients in whom sub-motor activity was stimulated. Repetitive low frequency TMS has shown promise in schizophrenia, with Lee and associates in 2005 reporting reduction in psychotic symptoms after a course of ten daily treatments in treatment-resistant cases, with side effects limited to fleeting headache and amnesia. Further research is needed, but findings suggest that prolonged low level stimulation may be a more effective mode of convulsive therapy than the sudden, generalised

25 Hoenig J, Lieberman DM (1953): 'The epileptic threshold in schizophrenia'. *Journal of Neurology*, Neurosurgery and Psychiatry, 16: 30–34.

action of ECT, and may explain the past superiority of insulin coma therapy. In another twist of serendipity, it has been noted that some patients exposed to the common diagnostic procedure of magnetic resonance imaging, who happened to be depressed, have returned home from their scan in raised spirits.

The relationship between epilepsy and functional psychosis leaves many unanswered questions. Both disorders are constructs of blurred demarcation. Epilepsy is straddled by several borderline states, while between bipolar disorder and schizophrenia is the nebulous intermediary of schizoaffective disorder, and the extent of overlap with functional psychoses has led to growing criticism of Kraepelin's classification. It is interesting that induced seizures are effective in treating severe depression, yet epidemiological studies have shown that depressive states are prominent in the psychiatric comorbidity of epilepsy (this may be partly an iatrogenic result of anticonvulsant medication). In his research on epilepsy in mental hospitals, TA Betts found in both chronic cases and new admissions that seizures were related to delusional behaviour, and inversely related to depression. Recent literature suggests that mania may be more common than thought in epilepsy, its frequency leading Dietrich Blumer to coin the term 'interictal dysphoric disorder'.[26] Anticonvulsants are increasingly used in affective disorders to supplement or replace lithium, and are often more effective in manic phases.[27] In 1971 in Japan, where lithium treatment was not yet available, Takezaki and Hanaoka found that carbamazepine, an anticonvulsant in use since the 1960s, controlled mania. For more than two decades this drug has been used as a second-line mood-stabilising treatment, and has shown value in various other non-epileptic conditions. Indeed, psychiatrist Jonathan Himmelhoch described carbamazepine as 'a drug in search of a disorder'.[28]

The possibility of a large sub-epileptic population with biological disturbance manifesting in mood swings is intriguing, and justifies concerted investigation by neurologists and psychiatrists of a syndrome absent from the disease taxonomies of brain and mind. Further research would enhance knowledge of the relationship between mood changes and epileptic or sub-epileptic activity. Environmental stress would be an important factor in this enquiry. Neuroscientist Michael Persinger of Laurentian University in Canada speculated that the temporal lobes may be sufficiently sensitive to fluctuations in the electromagnetic atmosphere to pro-

26 Blumer D (1997): 'Antidepressant and double antidepressant treatment for the affective disorder of epilepsy'. *Journal of Clinical Psychiatry*, 58: 3–11.

27 Barry JL, Lembke A, Huynh N (2001): 'Affective disorders in epilepsy'. In *Psychiatric Issues in Epilepsy: A Practical Guide to Diagnosis and Treatment* (eds AB Ettinger, AM Kanner). Philadelphia: Lippincott, Williams & Wilkins, 45–71.

28 Himmelhoch JM (1984): 'Major mood disorders and epileptic changes'. In *Psychiatric Aspects of Epilepsy* (ed. D Blumer). Washington: American Psychiatric Press, 271–291.

duce microseizures in otherwise healthy people. Whatever the mechanism, if an affective-epileptoid cyclical complex exists, the likelihood of some cases having a circalunar pattern would raise the possibility of entrainment, a tendency found in Winnifred Cutler's menstrual studies. Given the confounding effect of medication in patients with established epilepsy or bipolar affective disorder, naturalistic study of a subdiagnostic group would be justifiable.

From linear to systems thinking

In the hundred years since Kraepelin, psychiatry has neglected periodicity in mental disorder. This omission is explained by Thomas Wehr as 'the cultural shift from a cyclic to a linear perception of time, so that psychiatrists and patients may be more likely to perceive affective recurrences as a succession of separate events than as a seasonal cycle of events'.[29] The human being is objectified and compartmentalised by medicine, with little interest in the systemic interplay in which all organic life exists. Despite the unifying zeal of Einstein and his successors, and wider social and philosophical challenge to reductionism, the sciences continue to diverge like spokes of a wheel, each discipline moving further apart from its neighbours, with further subdivisions as new areas of knowledge and enquiry develop. Stuck in a groove of esotericism, psychiatrists have little common ground with physicists, and in consequence no theoretical framework has been established for investigating mental disorder within geophysical parameters.

To be fair, psychiatry is more eclectic than is portrayed by critics, but its armamentarium is primarily pharmaceutical, with mental disorder treated as a biochemical aberration. Internal fault is treated by internal corrective. Daniel Kirsch, current specialist in electromedicine, urged a change in outlook:

> Western universities are still teaching that life is based on a chemical model. Given the explosive growth in electrical technologies and our ever increasing understanding of physics, it is more realistic in the 21st century to view biological processes on an electrochemical basis.[30]

---

29 Wehr TA (1989): 'Seasonal affective disorder: a historical overview'. In *Seasonal Affective Disorders and Phototherapy* (eds Rosenthal NE, Blehar MC). New York: Guilford Press, 11–32.

30 Kirsch DL (2006): 'Why electromedicine? Harnessing the electrochemical basis of biological processes, electromedicine offers a wide rage of applications in the pain area'. *Practical Pain Management*, July/August: 52–54.

From the vitalist stance, life cannot be fully explained by the physical laws of nature, but whereas the aethereal concept is preserved in the Chinese *qi* and Ayurvedic *prana*, western medicine has long abandoned such metaphysics. Yet one does not need to be religious or a romanticist to believe that human experience and behaviour may be influenced by forces not yet understood. Prevailing scientific discourse remains Newtonian — linear, universal, determinist — as though relativity is an inconvenience. However, as controversial philosopher of science Paul Feyeraband argued, science has more in common with myth than most people realise; between occasional episodes of anarchy, it is a conservative enterprise in which dominant views are reinforced. The debate on global warming demonstrates how dissenting ideas are suppressed by the more powerful side, with sceptics refused funding and publication, and subjected to *ad hominem* attacks. Medicine is apt to eschew radical ideas in maintaining its epistemological mastery, but Robert Becker argued that a narrow empiricist dogma has precluded a deeper understanding of the *milieu* of health and illness:

> The gulf between folk therapy and our own stainless-steel version is illusory. Western medicine springs from the same roots and acts through the same little-understood forces as its country cousins. All worthwhile medical research and every medicine man's intuition is part of the same quest for knowledge of the same elusive healing energy.[31]

As complex and unpredictable phenomena, subtle energy fields have potentially diverse influences on health. Emphasising the therapeutic possibilities of environmental energy, Paul Rorsch, clinical professor at the American Institute of Stress, described how relatively weak forces can have massive impact:

> Resonance explains why singers can shatter a glass several feet away if the note they create is the same resonance frequency as the glass. The collapse of the Takoma suspension bridge at Puget Sound in 1940 was caused by wind-induced vibrations that were not particularly strong but just happened to coincide with the bridge's resonance frequency.[32]

Rorsch analogised our interrelating physiological systems to an orchestra, whose concerted performance relies on a conductor. Were the baton to direct an exogenous rhythm, the extent of environmental influence on biological and mental phenomena would require a radical overhaul in medical and psychiatric theory. Passing the stumbling block of disciplinary segregation requires systems thinking. This approach emerged in biology and engineering in the 1920s as a rebuttal of the linear cause-and-effect

---

31 Becker RO, Selden G (1985): *The Body Electric: Electromagnetism and the Foundation of Life*. New York: Harper, p29.
32 Rorsch PJ (2009): 'Bioelectromagnetic and subtle energy medicine: the interface between mind and matter'. *Annals of the New York Academy of Science*, 1172: 297–311.

model. An advocate of metadisciplinary science, Austro-Hungarian biologist Ludwig von Bertalanffy (1901–1972) devised his general systems theory in opposition to subject-object dualism and the prevailing determinism in his field.[33] He criticised the concept of homeostasis, originating in the work of French scientist Claude Bernard (1813–1878) and developed by Walter Bradford Cannon, as a narrow view of living things adapting passively to their surroundings. Equilibrium is indeed maintained through response to external stimuli such as temperature, but as von Bertalanffy observed, the dynamic relationship is not always appreciated: people are not only *affected by*, but also *affect* their environment — not only through physiological processes such as respiration, but also by free will. Biologists now accept that evolution is an interaction of organism and habitat. In tangible ways, we create our universe, but we are also tuned to natural rhythms of which we have only scratched the surface in understanding.

According to von Bertalanffy, equilibrium is a state only reached at death; the driving force of life and evolutionary development is stress. He argued that the greatest human achievements in science and the humanities are not the product of homeostatic tendency, but of *élan vital*. Such thinking built on the noumenal constructions of Kant and Arthur Schopenhauer (1788–1860), the latter philosopher having drawn a somewhat pessimistic picture of human existence in perpetual slavery to nature, but with escape to transcendental reality through art. Evidence that equilibrium is not the ultimate satisfaction of needs is in the higher incidence of psychological problems in affluent, democratic societies; paradoxically, lack of tension appears to correlate with anxiety.

Just as each living organism from fungus to human being alters the environment as well as vice versa, the systemic input of the Moon must be relatively enormous. Lunar cycles produce known effects at the macro-level of geophysical variables, but at the micro-level of *Homo sapiens*, we are unsure. An obstacle to understanding atmospheric and cosmic influences on health is the lack of systems thinking in medicine, which remains a conservative discipline, slow to embrace radical theories that threaten existing principles and practice. While the growth of chronobiology shows some advance from a conventional linear model, pioneer Jürgen Aschoff opposed the development of specialist journals and symposia, arguing that the study of rhythmic phenomena should permeate all biomedical science. If endogenous cyclicity is neglected, attention to extrinsic influences is even further behind. Just as the electrodynamic theory of Harold Saxton Burr and successors has had minimal impact on mainstream medicine, Arnold Lieber's thesis of biological rhythms was less disparaged than

33   von Bertalanffy, L (1950): 'An outline of general system theory'. *British Journal for the Philosophy of Science*, 1: 134–165.

ignored: here was a clinician stepping outside his professional domain. Psychiatrists and physicists rarely meet.

The works of Burr and von Bertalanffy have, however, influenced theoretical endeavour in nursing, a profession concerned more with care than cure. Martha E Rogers (1914–1994) was a polymath who headed the Division of Nursing at New York University from 1954 to 1975. Rogers was the first nurse to argue that her discipline should refer not only to the knowledge of medicine, sociology and psychology, but also to physics and astronomy. *The Science of Unitary Human Beings*, first appearing as a nursing manual in 1970, presented a novel approach to human behaviour and the nursing process.[34] Rejecting conceptual divisions of mind and matter, and of the patient into physical, psychological and social spheres, Rogers described the human being as an indivisible energy field, in dynamic interaction with the environment. Nurses often claim to provide holistic care, but here was holism in the true sense of the term. Health and illness are not dichotomous, but manifestations of the rhythmic fluctuations of life. Each person's energy field has a unique pattern, and for Rogers the role of the nurse was to help patients to synergise with their surroundings. The culture of American nursing may have been intellectually superior to that of Britain and Europe, but Rogers' model was too complex for the average nurse to comprehend, let alone apply in practice. Perhaps Rogers herself was in the wrong field at the wrong time. Tuning into cosmic forces would require a radical redirection of healthcare.

Nonetheless, systems thinking has been embraced to greater extent in other human sciences. A catalyst was Kurt Lewin in the 1940s. Dissatisfied with how psychologists isolated types of behaviour, thus losing sight of the overall picture, Lewin founded a school of social psychology in which person and environment were considered as an interaction. He believed that individuals, groups and organisations alike exist in a social force field, a system in tension whereby behaviour is a product of positive and negative forces. Lewin's quasi-mathematical formulation was criticised for its spurious precision and mechanistic orderliness, but his work had seminal influence in management and business studies. Organisations began to be studied not in isolation but as interdependent elements of an open system. A current proponent is Peter Senge at the Massachusetts Institute of Technology, whose best-selling management treatise *The Fifth Discipline* urges systems thinking in a modern commercial environment of increasing complexity. Another application is systemic family therapy, in which the psychologist focuses not on a deviant member but at the whole family unit.

---

34   Rogers ME (1970): *An Introduction to the Theoretical Basis of Nursing*. Philadelphia: FA Davis. p6.

Despite the efforts of a minority of scholars, systems thinking is often given mere lip service in health sciences. Control and expertise are threatened by the blurred boundaries of systems thinking; theoretically, everything is connected to everything else. Furthermore, systems exhibit chaotic tendency, and are thus unpredictable. Yet sequential patterns and long-term cycles may be discerned, to the extent that probabilistic theory may be generated; the dynamic complexity of weather forecasting, for example, is yielding to the power of sophisticated computerised modelling. Regarding the entire universe as an open system, philosopher of science David Bohm posited an implicate reality in which all phenomena are explications of an underlying schema.[35] This implies that no subject of interest should be studied outside its natural situation. However, researchers cannot all be theoretical physicists!

A systemic approach may be applied at the micro-level, with the unit of study narrowed to the individual case, and developed outwards from there. A shift in focus from generalisation to the person-environment interplay could be more fruitful in investigating the relationship between Moon and mind. Critics Rotton and Kelly argued that not only is lunar influence on geophysical variables such as the magnetic field, ions and extremely low frequency waves slight at most, it would also vary from one person to next. This would justify targeted investigation of individual susceptibility to environmental stimuli. Intensive case studies may yet illuminate patterns of lunar periodicity lost in large samples. Ways and means for future lunar research are the concern of the final chapter.

35   Bohm D (1980): *Wholeness and the Implicate Order*. London: Ark.

Nine

Reconciling mind and cosmos

There is more in the heavens and earth than in your philosophy

Hamlet, William Shakespeare

From the Pyramid Texts through Paracelsian medicine to Pink Floyd, the Moon has loomed large in our collective psyche. The legend of lunar influence pervades society, but is this merely a remnant of pre-Enlightenment thinking, to which we should apply Occam's razor? On being interviewed on BBC Radio 4, the author felt compelled to distance himself from mysticism, setting out his stall by stating that if the Moon did affect mental illness, psychiatrists would surely have noticed it by now. After all, research has failed to refute the null hypothesis in any of the behavioural variables studied; even if positive findings were accepted, they would not have any general implications for clinical practice. Yet the response at conferences and other gatherings where I have presented this work, suggests that the outright rejection of lunar influence by the professional orthodoxy is discordant with the experience of many clinicians and their clients.

Tyranny of aggregation

In considering the theory and evidence for lunar influence on behaviour, inequities in the prevailing knowledge of mental health and disorder must be acknowledged. Mental health nursing, the leading source of lunar belief among the professions, remains a weak player in the epistemological game. How many times does one read a newspaper report of research on or by mental health nurses? One reason is that the essence of nursing, despite the current doctrine of evidence-based practice, is not so much in applied science but in a therapeutic rapport, the practitioner's expertise developing over a career of helping people in all kinds of physical, psychological and social difficulties. Despite inculcation of scientific language in trainees, nursing discourse remains anecdotal.

In the 1990s, when managing one of the first mental health crisis services in Britain, the author routinely collated daily and monthly totals for helpline contacts, emergency visits and overnight stays on the office whiteboard, but fellow nurses and social workers showed little interest in the statistical reports of this novel venture. For practitioners this was extremely challenging work, and there was never a shortage of adventures to relate to colleagues, sometimes laced with dark humour. Visiting callers from across the socio-economic spectrum, one night the team might be negotiating access to a squalid drug den in the concrete underworld, the next to a flint-walled farmhouse on the Downs, guarded by a fearsome flock of geese. From the stageside in a theatre of despair, there were many profound experiences for which 'Wednesday – 1 visit' could not reflect.

Nursing continues to be seen as a practical pursuit, more about *doing* than *thinking*. When the author's enquiring mind spurred a career change into research, he was struck by the contrast in capacity between the professions. Whereas the nurse must leave practice to engage in research, psychologists and psychiatrists have dedicated study time in their working week, facilitating praxis (integration of theory and practice). Getting involved in studies and attending conferences is elementary to professional development for psychiatrists, but for nurses such activity is regarded as extramural. With their contribution to knowledge suppressed by a combination of social stratification and limited scientific interest, nurses mutter from the galleries that their work with patients is beyond experimental investigation and statistical measurement. Not surprisingly, nurses do not love numbers, but when they accuse psychiatry of reductionism the argument is often crude, with the medical model and positivism as straw men. Yet their scepticism towards blunt quantification of an inherently humanistic endeavour is justifiable.

Psychometric instruments are a boon to research on cognition and behaviour, but however well tested for validity and reliability, they provide only a proxy indicator of the phenomenon of interest. While his own analyses have been challenged, Arnold Lieber surely made a salient point in criticising the reliance on conventional scientific methods in studying the relationship between behaviour and the environment. To understand lunar influence on body and mind, we must not only consider the physical effects of the hypothetical causative agent, but also the subtleties of the individual human being, whose responses to external stimuli may be beneath the radar of clinical surveillance. A creative approach should traverse the arbitrary boundaries of disciplines, and the ontological chasm between natural science and humanistic knowledge.

Deterministic science does not recognise the immaterial mind; our thoughts and beliefs, often irrational and capricious, are what William James regarded as mere epiphenomena of an underlying physiology. Despite attempts at *rapprochement*, the philosophical dualism of scientific explanation and lived experience persists, as in the *res cogitans* and *res extensa* of Descartes. Psychology is the discipline most immersed in this conundrum: on one hand is the interpretation-free doctrine of the behaviourists; on the other the empirically elusive theories of mentation. Indeed, the human sciences were late entrants to the scientific community because they did not readily fulfil the Comtean standards of positivism. For psychology to make progress as a science, mental activity had to be as quantifiable as physical objects and forces. A guiding light was the great biometrician Francis Galton (1822–1911), who argued:

> General impressions are never to be trusted. Unfortunately when they are of long standing they become fixed rules of life, and assume a prescriptive right not to be questioned. Consequently those who are not accustomed to original enquiry entertain a hatred and a horror of statistics. They cannot endure the idea of submitting their sacred impressions to cold-blooded verification. But it is the triumph of scientific men to rise superior to such superstitions, to desire tests by which the value of beliefs may be ascertained, and to feel sufficiently masters of themselves to discard contemptuously whatever may be found untrue.[1]

Ironically, cold-blooded, contemptuous and masterful might be terms used for the founders of modern statistics in their involvement in eugenics, a movement built on the science of genetics, which required a moderated determinism of statistical probability. The successive trio of Galton, Pearson and Fisher was instrumental in promoting state control of the gene pool. In 1925 Karl Pearson, who occupied the Galton Chair of Eugenics at Cambridge University, launched the *Annals of Eugenics*. Gracing each edition was the above quote from Galton, which his disciple regarded as the finest words ever written in science. Statistical methodology has undoubtedly been a vehicle for the advancement of knowledge, but it can be dehumanising, as demonstrated by the Soviet Union, whose totalitarian leader Josef Stalin is credited with the dark insight: 'when one man dies it is a tragedy; when thousands die it is a *statistic*'.[2] Whether in tractor production figures or in casualty waiting times, in judging success by number, human experience is too easily disregarded in a tyranny of aggregation, which continues to distort the aims and outcomes of public services.[3] Meanwhile false numerical precision is repeatedly displayed in the

---

1   Galton F (1879): 'Generic images'. *Proceedings of the Royal Institution*, 9: 9.
2   Perper JA, Cina SJ (2010): *When Doctors Kill: Who, Why and How*. New York: Springer.
3   This term borrowed from the author's academic colleagues Bryan MacIntosh and Trevor Murralls.

research findings that fill space in newspaper columns, of which the conflicting reports of lunar influence are an example.

Psychologists built their professional prestige on their ability to quantify all aspects of human behaviour, as though their mantra were: *if it moves, measure it*. Statistical methods operationalise a research question, but cannot account for human agency; results show what happened,. but not what will happen in future. The folly of determinism has been demonstrated in economics. Geoffrey Hodgson (2009) attributed the global financial crisis of 2008 to an excessively mathematical orientation in his discipline; obsessed in algebraic models, experts lost sight of the social forces that govern markets. Back in the 1970s another economist, EF Schumacher, in his philosophical treatise *Guide for the Perplexed*, urged subversion of the conventional epistemological hierarchy to elevate lived experience over the materialism of basic science. Without taking account of how people think and feel, science presents a narrow representation of truth, and can be dangerously misleading. As Einstein warned in a sign hung in his office at Princeton University: 'Not everything that can be counted counts, and not everything that counts can be counted.'[4]

In recent times psychology has espoused a more eclectic approach, both in research and practice. The currently dominant cognitive behaviour therapy bridges the internal focus of psychotherapy with the external objectivity of behavioural theory, and is a legacy of the 'third way' of humanistic psychology founded in the 1950s by Abraham Maslow and Carl Rogers. This therapeutic model gave primacy to the client's unique perspective, and was heavily influenced by the phenomenologist philosophy of Edmund Husserl (1859–1938) and his successor Martin Heidegger (1889–1976). Emerging in the heyday of Freud, phenomenologists strove to understand consciousness through description and interpretation of each person's 'being in the world'. The assumed distinction between subject and object was rejected as dualistic error, all experiences being inextricably mental and physical. Having contempt for modern industrial society, Heidegger believed that people had lost the sense of being at one with nature; there was deeper thinking than science in his individualist conception of authenticity. The idea that 'being' is contextual and temporal was developed by Maurice Merleau-Ponty (1908–1961), who argued that there is no private consciousness, but a *milieu*. In his treatise on hermeneutics *Phenomenology of Perception* (1945), Merleau-Ponty opposed both empiricism and rationalism, of which the flaws were revealed by the character Meno in Plato's dialogues: how can you search for something you do not know exists, and if you find that thing, how can you know it is the

---

4   Quoted by Rorsch PJ (2009): 'Bioelectromagnetic and subtle energy medicine: the interface between mind and matter'. *Annals of the New York Academy of Science*, 1172: 297–311.

thing of which you are unaware? Furthermore, neither approach reflects how people see their world. For Merleau-Ponty a holistic interaction of subjective and objective phenomena provided an ontological basis for human science.

Phenomenology was mostly confined to philosophical debate until the radical zeitgeist of the 1960s, when academe became a breeding ground for neo-Marxist critical theory, feminism and racial politics, all of which highlighted the role of knowledge in preserving the status quo. Science, with its positivist orientation, was regarded by avant-garde philosophers such as Michel Foucault and deconstructionist Jacques Derrida as a technocratic conspiracy to dominate the masses. Inspired by phenomenology and the existentialism of Jean-Paul Sartre and Albert Camus, postmodern ideology encouraged a humanistic revival in social science. Sociologists moved away from blunt structuralism to consider behaviour as the product of interpretation. However, without a robust means of eliciting and explaining individual experience, the output of such enquiry could be criticised as anecdote in plural. Classic ethnographic accounts, such as Margaret Mead's study of tribal life in Samoa and Erving Goffman's analysis of the culture of a New York state mental institution, were strong in verisimilitude but lacked scientific rigour. Qualitative research was placed on a scientific footing in 1967 when Barney Glaser and Anselm Strauss devised the strategy of 'grounded theory', which entails theoretical sampling and constant comparative analysis. While sociologists got there first, psychologists have belatedly embraced qualitative methodology. Today, dissertations of clinical psychology trainees are commonly based on interpretative phenomenological analysis — without a P figure in sight.

In treating meanings and emotions as valid data, the human sciences are reflecting wider epistemological change. Materialist science was undermined in the early twentieth century by the twin developments of Einstein's relativity and quantum mechanics, and the new physics led to the critical realist philosophy of Karl Popper.[5] In his *Logic of Scientific Discovery* in 1934, Popper subverted verificationism, arguing that no theory is valid unless it is possible for it to be falsified. As no irrefutable laws are attainable, we might come close to objective reality, but never actually arrive. Science may be the most reliable form of knowledge, but offers no final truth. Popper's writings became widely influential in the 1960s, when scientific absolutism was challenged from another angle. Thomas Kuhn

---

5   Einstein's theory of relativity does not state that everything is relative: while space, time and mass are relative to the observer, there is constancy in the speed of light. However, Einstein emphasised that the scientist is inextricable from the system being studied, while quantum theorists explained that the act of observing alters whatever is being observed.

described a revolutionary rather than evolutionary trajectory of knowledge, whereby all research and theory is framed by a prevailing paradigm, which is eventually overturned by a radical thesis or discovery, creating a new paradigm. For example, geocentrism was supplanted by the Copernican system, and Newtonian physics by relativity. Science, like consciousness, can only be understood in context.

Although the physical sciences did not follow the social strands of the human sciences in their lurch from naïve realism to multiple truths, the impact of philosophical and social critique threatened the status of scientific objectivity, as described by Robert Solomon:

> The conception of 'science' was constricted almost to the point of suffocation by the positivism of the thirties and relativised in the sixties to the point where the best theoreticians of science had lost their grasp of any clear-cut criterion that would distinguish astronomy from astrology or electromagnetic field theory from witchcraft and ESP.[6]

By limiting reality to individual perspective, relativism soon transpired as an intellectual *cul de sac*. In the phenomenological doctrine, the aforementioned observation by Berzelius of his lunar-regulated migraine would have to be accepted as true for him, and therefore real. Indeed, if someone adamantly believes in a full moon effect, no geophysical stimuli would be necessary. This is ontological nihilism: without generalisation, social science would be an oxymoron. Increasingly, researchers apply a mixture of quantitative and qualitative methods, but while an eclectic definition of science appears to blur the boundary between empiric and aesthetic phenomena, the underlying ontological debate may never reach a satisfactory conclusion. As the most trusted route to knowledge, the method of natural science continues to dominate research.

Heroic psychiatry

In his *Birth of the Clinic*, Foucault told how science is used as an instrument of medical hegemony, placing body and mind beyond the lay domain. Windows to esoteric knowledge have opened in the internet era, yet credentialism prevails: an outsider may have access to information, but only through a professional framework can it be properly understood and applied. While researchers are increasingly combining quantitative and qualitative methods, thus blurring the boundaries between empiric and

6 Solomon RC (1993): *The Passions: Emotions and the Meaning of Life*. Indianapolis: Hackett, pp78–79.

aesthetic phenomena, the underlying ontological debate may never be resolved. Quantification of healthcare has had additional impetus since the 1970s, when Archie Cochrane presented his manifesto for evidence-based medicine. The Cochrane Collaboration, an international body for systematic review of research on health interventions, places randomised controlled trials atop its hierarchy of evidence, with the non-experimental descriptive study just above the bottom rung of anecdotal report. Deep insights into a person's 'being in the world' have no place in Cochrane's 'gold standard' research.

For all the achievements of medical science, sometimes exaggerated credit is given to the white coats of laboratory and clinic. Steadily increasing longevity over the last hundred years is not so much due to medicine, as commonly believed, but to general improvements in living conditions. Furthermore, excessive clinical encroachment on people's lives can be harmful, a case argued most emphatically by Ivan Illich in 1976 in his treatise on iatrogenic medicine. Doctors may cure or alleviate illness, but health is a product of hereditary, social and environmental circumstances, and in a democracy it is society and its elected politicians who are responsible for creating the optimal conditions for well being. If medicine were the principal determinant of life expectancy, it would also be responsible for all socio-demographic inequalities in mortality. This would be unreasonable, not least because in practice the profession has concerned itself rather less with prevention than with treatment. Asklepius trumps Hygeia.

Heroic assumptions are also made about the technological feats of psychiatry, where scientific discipline has been a corrective against popular but unfounded beliefs about the mind and the mad. In their book *The Great Ideas of Clinical Science*, psychologists O'Donahue, Lilienfeld and Fowler gave as an example the traditional idea 'that human physiology was a function of the Moon'. After remarking on how practitioners are as prone as the lay person to confirmation bias, illusory correlation and erroneous causal beliefs, the authors committed themselves to a slanted narrative of psychiatric progress:

> In the first world, few if any mental hospitals can today be called 'snake pits'. However, before the rise of effective antipsychotic medications in the 1950s, the situation was far different. The delusions and hallucinations of individuals with schizophrenia were so unmanageable that patients were put in cells, chained to chairs, or, if not controlled, yelling and spreading their faeces on the walls.[7]

Historians of psychiatry would refute this simplistic notion of psychopharmacology rescuing the mental patient. There was plenty of

---

7   O'Donahue WT, Lilienfeld SO, Fowler KA (2007): 'Science is an essential safeguard against human error'. In *The Great Ideas of Clinical Science: 17 Principles that every Mental Health Professional should Understand* (eds Lilenfeld SO, O'Donahue WT). New York: Routledge. 1–27, p5.

evidence that tranquillisers alleviated symptoms and enabled earlier discharge, but as explained in Chapter 5, the social forces of change were already at work in the psychiatric institutions. Nonetheless, the Largactil story became accepted as the singular means of the unlocking of the mental hospital.

Statistically significant but spurious results; lack of solid theoretical foundation; researchers finding what they seek; publication bias; conflicting effects—such criticisms of studies reporting lunar correlation could just as reasonably be aimed at the established evidence base of psychiatry. To illustrate, let us consider the scientific basis of antidepressant medication. While the author knows personally and professionally people who have found antidepressants a godsend, investigation by experts such as psychiatrist David Healy and psychologist Irving Kirsch suggest that the number of patients genuinely benefiting from the chemical mechanism may be much lower than 'Big Pharma' would admit. Analysing data from antidepressant drug trials submitted to the FDA (the American licensing body for pharmaceutical products), Kirsch and colleagues found an overall mean difference between drug and placebo of less than two points on the Hamilton Rating Scale for Depression—a clinically insignificant result. The reporting of antidepressant effectiveness (for example, in the World Health Organisation manual on psychiatric disorder) focuses on the two-thirds of patients who responded positively in trials, but this ignores the improvement found in the control group—as if the 'C' in RCT does not exist.

Overstated antidepressant efficacy has been exposed by researchers using freedom of information law to obtain full data sets from pharmaceutical companies. A review by Turner and associates showed that almost a third of seventy-four clinical trials registered by the FDA were not published.[8] Of thirty-eight trials producing positive results, thirty-seven were published; of thirty-six trials with negative or dubious results, twenty-two did not reach print. Moreover, in the fourteen studies deemed by the authors to show little or no therapeutic benefit, eleven were presented with positive conclusions. Consequently, 94 per cent of trials were positive! This is a major issue because practice guidelines are based on peer-reviewed literature. Yet the published findings alone should cast sufficient doubts, with a lack of dose-response relationship, and little evidence that antidepressants reduce suicide risk any more than placebo. Furthermore, the presumed neurotransmitter mechanism for antidepressants has been challenged. Kirsch noted that trials of tianeptine, a recently introduced drug, showed a response rate equivalent to other antidepressants, but its action is opposite—it *suppresses* serotonin. This is surely no

8   Turner EH, Matthews AM, Linardatos E, Tell RA, Rosenthal R (2008): 'Selective publication of antidepressant trials and its influence on apparent efficacy'. *New England Journal of Medicine*, 358: 252–260.

more logical than the inconsistent temporal patterns reported by research-ers of lunar influence.

Near equipotency would suggest a strong placebo effect, but as depres-sion is normally self-remitting, recoveries would occur in both active and placebo groups irrespective of beliefs about treatment. The small statisti-cal superiority of antidepressants over placebo was described as 'a meth-odological artefact' by critical psychiatrist Joanne Moncrieff. Trials tend to favour the active drug because the standard procedure of double blinding is undermined by the appearance of side effects, compounding expectancy bias in practitioner and patient. Having only modest advantage over pla-cebo, while causing side effects and withdrawal symptoms, antidepres-sants have dubious cost-effectiveness, yet the number of prescriptions continues to rise steadily. A classic marketing success perhaps, but that would only partly explain, because as Gary Greenberg described in his polemic *Manufacturing Depression*, psychiatrists are heavily invested in the schema of 'magic bullets'.[9] The psychiatrist plays the role of professional expert and receives status affirmation from the patient, who is relieved by medical diagnosis and treatment. The 'consulting room game' is an illus-tration of the transactional analysis founded by social psychologist Eric Berne (1910–1970), who defined interaction as 'an ongoing series of com-plementary ulterior transactions progressing to a well-defined predictable outcome'.[10] Psychiatric practice is inextricable from social dynamics.

For all its scientific safeguards, the hypothetico-deductive model can produce anomalous evidence, but treatments are sometimes prescibed despite contrary research findings. State purseholders and insurance com-panies try to limit treatment options, but doctors have professional auton-omy and to some extent they can sidestep disagreeable policies or research evidence. Indeed, health service administration is a compromise between management and the powerful medical profession, and doctors continue to work above rather than alongside other clinicians. In mental health ser-vices, while psychiatrists have embraced multidisciplinary teamwork, psychologist Lucy Johnstone in her book *Users and Abusers of Psychiatry* described various controlling tactics, which include: ignoring or discount-ing non-medical input; attributing all improvement to medical interven-tion; dismissing counter-evidence to prevailing practice; selectively quoting research findings as the definitive truth; and regarding behaviour as diagnostic features rather than as a meaningful response to events.[11] The old hospital hierarchy has gone, but with psychiatrists retaining clinical leadership, the perspectives of lower-status but experientially

9   Greenberg G (2010): *Manufacturing Depression: The Secret History of a Modern Disease.* London: Bloomsbury.

10   Berne E (1964): *Games People Play*. Harmondsworth: Penguin.

11   Johnstone L (2000): *Users and Abusers of Psychiatry*. London: Routledge.

enriched workers are confined to a bracketed level of knowledge. With nurses at considerable disadvantage in contributing to theory and evidence, it is all the more important that psychiatrists should be receptive to despatches from the frontline. Within reason, any observation of fellow clinicians is potentially worthy of further investigation. Through a Foucauldian lens, the insights of nurses are on the wrong side of a professional knowledge barrier. The anecdotalism of nursing, the statistically-precise empiricism of psychology, the biologically-orientated practice of psychiatry — each has something to offer as a source of mental health knowledge.

A way forward

To date, the lunar hypothesis has been investigated within a narrow epistemology, with data on admissions to psychiatric hospital, suicides, violent incidents and crisis calls providing an unsatisfactory answer to the fundamental question of whether Moon affects mind. Analysis has progressed from simple correlational techniques, but it is possible for interesting temporal signals to be missed by sophisticated methods such as time series analysis because people may respond (directly or indirectly) to different points on the lunar cycle. For example, if 80 per cent of a sample is immune to a lunar effect, and the remaining 20 per cent are affected in equal proportions at each quarter phase, no correlation would be found. A zero sum would also result if lunar position affected roughly similar numbers of subjects in opposite ways. In his review Salvatore Garzino remarked that research on lunar and cosmic influence on behaviour is at a stage no more advanced than that of psychology in the nineteenth century.

Ambiguity from over fifty years of research output is likely to continue until the development of a conceptual framework of specified behaviours and population at risk. Instead of relying on quantitative analysis, researchers should engage with the phenomenon at a higher level of intensity. Strangely, the growth of qualitative research in healthcare literature has not been reflected in studies of lunar influence, despite its widely accepted value in exploratory investigation. Since grounded theory was introduced by Glaser and Strauss, a principle of qualitative research has been that any theory generated must take account of every case, however deviant or extreme (this contrasts with statistical methods, where outliers may be excluded from analysis). If lunar influence has noticeable effects in only a small fraction of the populace, researchers should not dilute or delete unusual instances, but strive to explain how and why these differ from the norm.

Tom, a community mental health nurse and ex-colleague of the author, told of a patient he has been seeing lately, who is certain that the peaks and troughs of her moods correspond with the phases of the Moon. Her belief may be erroneous, and would be more likely to raise her psychiatrist's eyebrows than an application for research funding, but perhaps cases like this deserve closer attention. Major medical discoveries have arisen from single observations. In 1907 German psychiatrist Alois Alzheimer (1864–1915) identified the eponymous type of dementia from postmortem investigation of a middle-aged woman who had displayed cognitive impairment normally found in senile dementia; her condition was not a natural consequence of ageing, but a distinct neuropathology. Perhaps the most famous investigator of individual cases was the Viennese neurologist Sigmund Freud, whose revelations on the unconscious workings of the mind arose from intensive analysis. Detailed investigations of lunar cases were conducted in the past by Leonard Ravitz, and there are lessons to be drawn from the strengths and weaknesses of this presentation.[12]

Free from restriction to a priori variables, case studies can contribute in various ways to knowledge, by casting doubt on the generalisability of existing theory, and as a heuristic primer to theoretical development in rare or poorly understood phenomena. Case studies may be criticised for lack of rigour and generalisability, and caveats should be issued. Individual observations cannot be considered as evidence of causation, and are no substitute for conventional methods of scientific investigation; bias is a danger when drawing conclusions from a single pattern of events, and the researcher must not allow initial impressions to develop into circular reasoning. An important point about case studies is that the researcher is not simply telling a story, although this may be fascinating by itself. Meaningfulness is not so much in what is unique about the person, but in generalisable concepts. Robert Yin, expert on case study methodology, likened the role to that of a detective, finding clues by sifting through reams of data that would overwhelm the undisciplined reader.[13] Although a case study is an open-ended enquiry, a theoretical perspective should run through the investigation, guiding the process from initial idea to conclusions (even with the optimally open approach of grounded theory, Glaser and Strauss reminded researchers of the need for theoretical direction). Rather than a top-down deductive approach of testing the hypothesis in specified sub-groups, an inductive approach would work upwards from individual people with suspected perilunar patterns.

12   Ravitz (1962). Available online.
13   Robert K Yin (1994): *Case Study Research: Design and Methods* (2nd edition). Thousand Oaks, California: Sage.

Unusually for clinical research, almost all studies of lunar influence have been retrospective. A rare exception was the prospective investigation of sleep and lunar cycles by Röösli and associates (see Chapter 7), in which participants were blinded from the purpose of the study. Scientific scepticism towards self-report measures, particularly of a suggestive phenomenon, is understandable. However, it would be neither ethical nor valid to conduct an entire research programme on masked intent. Concern about bias should not constrain exploratory zeal, and scientists should be less cynical towards subjective experience as a valid basis for knowledge. To illustrate the limits of retrospective quantification, consider the common idea that dreams are more vivid on nights of full moon (an observation I made myself as a teenager, albeit without any attempt at verification). Multiple factors influence dreams, including recent or imminent events, relationships, and consumption of caffeine, alcohol or other drugs. Atmospheric variables such as humidity may also hold sway, and it is not inconceivable that the Moon could also play a role in our nocturnal drama. EEG can provide objective measurement of electrical waves indicative of dream activity, but a really meaningful study would explore the content and intensity of dreams as reported by the participant, in diaries or questionnaires.

To accept information from the potentially biased source of the research participant should be no more anathema than it is in clinical assessment. Indeed, a discipline with a long tradition of combining objective information with subjective human experience is psychiatry, which traverses the Cartesian division of mind and matter. Existentialist Karl Jaspers, professor of psychiatry (1916–1922) and philosophy (1922–1937) at Heidelberg, described the practitioner's dual role of *Verstehen* (understanding) and *Erklären* (explanation); the former to elicit a unique narrative, the latter relating to general theory. Arguing that scientific knowledge had been erroneously defined by the premises of natural science, Jaspers claimed that no case could ever be comprehended by a single method, and that enquiry into individual experiences could be as scientific as measuring behaviour across a large sample. A patient can be *known* not by diagnostic category but by eliciting the unique individual experience and behaviour in its particular context.

Jaspers was writing in the interwar years, when Freudian theory had as much influence on the *Nervenklinik* as did Kraepelin. Sadly, Adolph Meyer's psychiatry of 'reaction types', whereby mental disorder was understood as an individual response to adversity, has long been abandoned by a profession that has pursued objectivity at all costs. The ascent of neo-Kraepelinian psychiatry since the 1970s, spurred by widely publicised reports of diagnostic inconsistencies and the Rosenhan scandal, is reflected by the descriptive but atheoretical DSM classification, to which pharmaceutical agents are targeted. Psychiatric conditions, while presented as discrete clinical entities, are rather arbitrarily defined constructs with circularity of symptoms and diseases. The inner world of the patient is irrelevant to diagnostic instruments and biochemical intervention. Unique and apparently relevant experiences (such as the interesting periodicity in Tom's patient) are likely to be ignored, because they are not listed on the diagnostic menu and therefore do not contribute to the treatment plan.

While often accused of biomedical dogmatism, in practice psychiatrists do take a broad view of the patient's situation in formulating a diagnosis and treatment plan. An eclectic approach is becoming more evident in the psychiatric literature, with the most stuffy journals now accepting qualitative research papers. As in other fields of knowledge, bridges are being built between positivist and phenomenological paradigms. This 'third movement' in human science has philosophical roots in the pragmatism of Charles Sanders Peirce (1839–1914) and John Dewey (1859–1952), in whose New World optimism, knowledge was the vehicle for the betterment of society. Peirce rejected the dualism of 'knowing' and 'reality', defining truth as socially accepted knowledge. Eschewing metaphysical debate, Dewey argued that methods should be judged by their capacity for providing useful information. While methodological pluralism offers the best of both worlds, its theoretical basis is contestable. As qualitative methodologists Guba and Lincoln argued, the two paradigms are of diametrically opposed ontology: one approach posits objective reality while the other denies it. However, this may be a false dichotomy. Wherever it starts, all research rotates in a cycle of ideas and data, progressing from observations to inferences through inductive logic, and from hypotheses to observations through deductive reasoning. Furthermore, we must acknowledge that many of the most imaginative discoveries in the history of science arose not from disciplined enquiry, but from chance observations — often by lay people unrestrained by scientific rules of engagement.

Pragmatism, however, is not always a force for the good. Older psychiatrists such as Professor Alastair Macdonald at the Institute of Psychiatry in London fear for the future of the specialty. Worsening recruitment problems, according to Alastair, can be attributed to the traditionally humanistic bent of psychiatry being suppressed by homogenisation and biological pre-occupation, which reduce the need for understanding and interpretation of the patient as a fellow human being.[14] Diagnosis is not so straightforward as reading from a menu of symptoms, but standardisation has perhaps made idiosyncrasies less relevant to the process of assessment and treatment. The patient is mapped on to a diagnostic category, and

14 Personal communication.

treated accordingly. If somebody complained of mood shifts on a four-weekly frequency, a possible menstrual cause might be investigated, but should the Moon be mentioned as a possible factor, this would be side-stepped if not dismissed. Even if such attribution had some temporal if not causative evidence, there is no value to such information in the treatment plan. A daily pill will do the trick: no more cycles — lunar or otherwise.

The hardened scientist of the positivist mould would recoil from an evidence base built on subjective experience with its attendant bias and limited generalisability, but perhaps sceptics waiting for numerical evidence would be impressed by this study conducted in the most quantified environment of all — the stock market. According to the *Financial Times*, technical analysts at the Royal Bank of Scotland examined the performance of six major indices (FTSE 100, S & P 500, Dax, EuroStoxx 50, Hang Seng and CAC40) in relation to lunar cycles.[15] Compared to the long-term daily average, activity on the days of new and full moon was relatively volatile. For example, the mean change in FTSE 100 value since 1986 was 0.55 points (0.02 per cent), but 5.17 points (0.11 per cent) at new moon, and 6.42 points (0.13 per cent) at full moon. This suggests potential financial gain in trading on new and full moon days. The RBS team found that if an investor, beginning with £1,000, had traded only twice a month since 1984, buying shares at new moon and selling at full moon, the product would have been £12,116 (a profit of £11,116). If however the timing had been reversed (buying at full moon), the investor would have reaped merely £2,036. Investing the £1,000 without selling would have amassed £5,130. Based on records from 1928 to 2010, a lunar trading strategy in the S & P 500 would have been even more profitable. Soberly, reporter Merryn Somerset Webb remarked that this finding was unlikely to be exploited, as transaction and index fund management fees would deter the frequency of trading necessary to achieve a bonus. Nonetheless, the report shows that the pin-striped stockbroker may be as sensitive to the Moon as the stereotypical mental patient. What was on investors' minds as they contributed to this lunar market?

Conclusion

Lunacy has fared badly in an epistemological context of heroic medicine, and an evidence-based doctrine built on exaggerated faith in statistics. The vital spirit, anthropocentrism and other romantic ideas have been aban-

15   Webb MS (2010): 'Looney, lunar or simply moonstruck?' *Financial Times*, 10/11 July.

doned to the ignorant past. And yet just as Socrates remarked that the more he learned, the less he knew, modern science finds unremitting challenges beyond its materialist tradition. While each new discovery may seem to bring us closer to mastering the universe (or universes), the goalposts are continually moving. Just as the fallibility of logic is demonstrated by self-referential paradox, positivism is teased by chaos in the system – in the dance of the electron, or in the free will of scientists themselves. Recalling the emphasis on doubt by the Sceptic philosophers of ancient Greece, science may be described as a process of organised scepticism. Proof proceeds from premises based on assumptions for which no proof is provided. Researchers claiming to have confirmed or refuted the lunar hypothesis have done no such thing – they have merely measured correlation between chosen variables in a chosen context. Disbelieving reviewers have asserted that the burden of proof lies with the believers, but surely a more trustworthy enquiry would be conducted by open-minded but methodical researchers who are prepared to overcome professional prejudice to examine a phenomenon that is both preposterous and possible.

Beans spurt, sea urchins bulge, worms glow, clams open, wolves howl. What theoretical obstacle precludes human sensitivity to the perturbations of our satellite? Common sense and experience tell us that the Moon cannot have great impact on our lives, and even the research findings of lunar correlation are not suggestive of much practical or clinical import. However, the topic continues to attract researchers across the world, with an endless stream of papers on lunar influence on all kinds of biological, mental and social phenomena. No report should be accepted without scrutiny, but it would be reasonable to state that published studies have generally been conducted as systematic investigations from the stance of objective empiricism, complying with modern standards of statistical analysis. Most scientific and professional journals with reputations to maintain would simply reject offerings on the interference of the Moon based on obviously flawed data collection or analysis. One cannot say with confidence that the Moon is responsible for the temporal patterns observed by researchers, but coincidental connections justify further investigation. Sceptics will argue that many studies have refuted a lunar effect, but from the ambiguity of findings overall, it is clear that the entire methodology and theoretical framework remains at a basic stage of development. It may disappoint some readers that this book does not provide any definitive answers to the lunar question, but it has at least presented an argument for further research. On the basis of evidence to date, it is too early to put the Moon to bed.

Bibliography

Abell GO, Singer B (eds 1981): *Science and the Paranormal*. New York: Scribner.

Adderley EE, Bowen GW (1962): 'Lunar component in precipitation data'. *Science*, 137: 749–750.

Addison J (1712): *Ode*. Retrieved from www.bible-researcher.com.

Al-Khalili J (2010): *Pathfinders: the Golden Age of Arabic Science*. London: Allen Lane.

Almond B (1988): *Philosophy*. Harmondsworth: Penguin.

Amaddeo F, Bisoffi G, Micciolo R, Piccinelli M, Tansella M (1997): 'Frequency of contact with community-based psychiatric services and the lunar cycle: a 10-year case study'. *Social Psychiatry and Psychiatric Epidemiology*, 32: 323–326.

American Psychiatric Association (1980): *Diagnostic and Statistical Manual of Mental Disorders* (3rd edition). Washington, DC: American Psychiatric Association.

American Psychiatric Association (1987): *Diagnostic and Statistical Manual of Mental Disorders* (3rd edition, revised). Washington, DC: American Psychiatric Association.

Anonymous (1850): *Familiar Views of Lunacy and Lunatic Life: With Hints on the Personal Care and Management of Those who are Afflicted with Temporary or Permanent Derangement*. London: John W Parker.

Arrhenius S (1898): 'Die Einwirkung kosmische Einflüsse auf physiologische Verhältnisse'. *Skandinavisches Archiv für Physiologie*, 8: 367–416.

Baker RR (1981): 'Man and other vertebra: a common perspective to migration and navigation'. In *Animal Migration* (ed DJ Aidley). Cambridge: Cambridge University Press. 241-260.

Balling RC, Cerveny RS (1995): Influence of lunar phase on daily global temperatures. *Science*, 267: 1481-1483.

Barham GF (1907): 'Notes on the management and treatment of the epileptic insane with special reference to the NaCl-free (or hypochlorination) diet'. *Journal of Mental Science*, 53: 361–367.

Barr W (2000): 'Lunacy revisited: the influence of the moon on mental health and quality of life'. *Journal of Psychosocial Nursing and Mental Health Services*, 38: 28-35.

Barry JL, Lembke A, Huynh N (2001): 'Affective disorders in epilepsy'. In *Psychiatric Issues in Epilepsy: A Practical Guide to Diagnosis and Treatment* (eds AB Ettinger, AM Kanner). Philadelphia: Lippincott, Williams & Wilkins. 45-71.

Bauer SF, Hornick EJ (1968): 'Lunar effect on mental illness: the relationship of moon phase to psychiatric emergencies'. *American Journal of Psychiatry*, 125: 696–697.

Baxendale S, Fisher J (2008): 'Moonstruck? The effect of the lunar cycle on seizures'. *Epilepsy and Behavior*, 13: 549–550.

Becker RO (1972): 'Electromagnetic forces and life processes'. *Technology Review*, 75: 2–8.

Becker RO, Selden G (1985): *The Body Electric: Electromagnetism and the Foundation of Life*. New York: Harper.

Bell B, Defouw R (1966): 'Dependence of the lunar modulation of geomagnetic activity on the celestial latitude of the moon'. *Journal of Geophysical Research*, 71: 951–957.

Benbadis SR, Chang S, Hunter J, Wang W (2004): 'The influence of the full moon on seizure frequency: myth or reality?' *Epilepsy and Behavior*, 5: 596–597.

Berger PL (1970): *A Rumour of Angels: Modern Society and the Rediscovery of the Supernatural*. Harmondsworth: Penguin.

Berger PL, Berger B, Kellner H (1974): *The Homeless Mind: Modernization and Consciousness*. Harmondsworth: Penguin.

Berne E (1964): *Games People Play*. Harmondsworth: Penguin.

Berrios GE (1979): 'Insanity and epilepsy in the nineteenth century'. In *Psychiatry, Genetics and Pathography: a Tribute to Eliot Slater* (eds M Roth, V Cowie). London: Gaskell.

Berrios GE (2004): 'Of mania: introduction'. *History of Psychiatry*, 15: 105–124.

Betts TA (1981): 'Epilepsy and the mental hospital'. In *Epilepsy and Psychiatry* (eds EH Reynolds, MR Trimble). Edinburgh: Churchill Livingstone. 175–184.

Bhattacharjee C, Bradley P, Smith M, Scally AJ, Wilson BJ (2000): 'Do animals bite more during a full moon? Retrospective observational analysis'. *British Medical Journal*, 321: 1559–1560.

Biermann T, Asemann R, McAuliffe C, Ströbel A, Keller J, Sperling W, Bleich S, Kornhuber J, Reulbach U (2009): 'Relationship between lunar phases and serious crimes of battery: a population-based study'. *Comprehensive Psychiatry*, 50: 573–577.

Blackburn S (1994): *The Oxford Dictionary of Philosophy*. Oxford: Oxford University Press.

Blackman S, Catalina D (1973): 'The moon and the emergency room'. *Perceptual and Motor Skills*, 37: 624–626.

Blackstone W (1765): *Commentaries on the Laws of England*. Oxford: Clarendon Press.

Blumer D (1997): 'Antidepressant and double antidepressant treatment for the affective disorder of epilepsy'. *Journal of Clinical Psychiatry*, 58: 3–11.

Bohm D (1980): *Wholeness and the Implicate Order*. London: Ark.

Bradley DA, Woodbury MA, Brier GW (1962): 'Lunar synodical period and widespread precipitation'. *Science*, 137: 748–749.

Bronowski J (1951): *The Common Sense of Science*. London: Heinemann.

Bronowski J (1977): *The Ascent of Man*. London: Book Club Associates.

Brown FA (1976): 'Biological clocks: endogenous cycles synchronized by subtle geophysical rhythms'. *Biosystems*, 8: 67–81.

Browning DC (1956): *Everyman's English Dictionary*. London: JM Dent & Sons.

Brzezinski A (1997): 'Melatonin in humans'. *New England Journal of Medicine*, 336: 186–195.

Bucknill JC, Tuke DH (1858): *A Manual of Psychological Medicine.* London: J & A Churchill.

Burr HS, Northrop FSC (1935): 'The electro-dynamic theory of life'. *Quarterly Review of Biology,* 10: 322–333.

Burrows GM (1828): *Commentaries on the Causes, Forms, Symptoms, and Treatment, Moral and Medical, of Insanity.* London: Thomas & George Underwood.

Busfield J (1986): *Managing Madness: Changing Ideas and Practice.* London: Hutchinson.

Butterfield H (1931): *The Whig Interpretation of History.* London: Bell.

Cade JF (1949): 'Lithium salts in the treatment of psychotic excitement'. *Medical Journal of Australia,* 2: 349–352.

Campbell DE, Beets JL (1978): 'Lunacy and the moon'. *Psychological Bulletin,* 85: 1123–1129.

Campbell D.E. (1982): 'Lunar-lunacy research: when enough is enough'. *Environment and Behavior,* 14: 418–424.

Campion N (2006): 'Astrology'. In *Encyclopedia of Witchcraft: the Western Tradition* (ed. RM Golden). Santa Barbara, California: ABC-CLIO. 64–65.

Camuffo D (2001): 'Lunar influences on climate'. *Earth, Moon and Planets,* 85–86: 99–113.

Carson R (1965): *The Sea.* London: Readers Union.

Cashford J (2004): *The Moon: Myth and Transformation.* Lecture to the Analytical Psychology Club, London. Retrieved from www. goddessreligion.pbworks.com.

Chandrasekhar S (1995): *Newton's Principia for the Common Reader.* Oxford: Oxford University Press.

Chapman A (1979): 'Astrological medicine'. In *Health, Medicine and Mortality in the Sixteenth Century* (ed. C Webster). Cambridge: Cambridge University Press. 275–300.

Chapman LJ (1961): 'A search for lunacy'. *Journal of Nervous and Mental Disease,* 132: 171–174.

Cheyne G (1734): *The English Malady, or a Treatise on Nervous Diseases of All Kinds.* London: Strahan & Leake.

Clark K (1969/1999): *Civilisation: A Personal View.* London: Folio Society.

Chudler EH (2007): 'The power of the full moon. Running on empty?' In *Tall Tales about the Mind and Brain: Separating Fact from Fiction* (ed. S Dellasalla). Oxford: Oxford University Press. 401–410.

Chung MC, Nolan P (1994): 'The influence of positivistic thought on nineteenth century nursing'. *Journal of Advanced Nursing,* 19: 226–232.

Climent CE, Plutchik R (1977): 'Lunar madness: an empirical study'. *Comprehensive Psychiatry,* 18: 369–374.

Cohen R (2010): *Chasing the Sun: the Epic Story of the Star that Gives Us Life.* London: Simon & Schuster.

Coones P (1983): 'The geographical significance of Plutarch's dialogue, *Concerning the Face which Appears on the Orb of the Moon'. Transactions of the Institute of British Geographers,* 8: 361–372.

Coxe JR (1817): *The Philadelphia Medical Dictionary* (2nd edition). Philadelphia: Thomas Dobson & Son.

Crammer JL (1959): 'Periodic psychoses'. *British Medical Journal,* i: 545–549.

Culpitt D (1976): *The Worlds of Science and Religion.* London: Sheldon Press.

Culver R, Rotton J, Kelly IW (1988): 'Moon mechanisms and myths: a critical appraisal of explorations of purported lunar effects on human behavior'. *Psychological Reports*, 62: 683–710.

Cutler WB (1980): 'Lunar and menstrual phase locking'. *American Journal of Obstetrics and Gynecology*, 137: 834–840.

Cutler WB, Schleidt WM, Freidmann E, Preti G, Stine R (1987): 'Lunar influences on the reproductive cycle in women'. *Human Biology*, 59: 959–972.

Cyr JJ, Kalpin RA (1987): 'The lunar-lunacy relationship: a poorly evaluated hypothesis'. *Psychological Reports*, 61: 391–400.

Danzl DF (1987): 'Lunacy'. *Journal of Emergency Medicine*, 5: 91–95.

Darwin C (1859): *On the Origin of Species by Means of Natural Selection, or the Preservation of Favoured Races in the Struggle for Life.* London: John Murray.

Darwin C (1871): *The Descent of Man.* London: John Murray.

Descartes R (1637/1971): *Discourse on the Method of Rightly Conducting One's Reason and of Seeking Truth in the Sciences* (translated GE Anscombe, P Geach). London: NUP.

Dekker T, Ford J, Rowley W (1658/1988): *The Witch of Edmonton.* London: Heinemann.

De Voge SD, Mikawa JK (1977): 'Moon phases and crisis calls: a spurious relationship'. *Psychological Reports*, 40: 387–390.

Dingman HF, Cleland CC, Swartz JD (1970): 'Institutional "wisdom" as expressed through folklore'. *Mental Retardation*, 8: 2–8.

Donne J (1624/ 1979): 'Meditation XVII'. In *The Norton Anthology of English Literature: Volume One* (4th edition, ed. MH Abrams). New York: Norton & Co.

Dosa D (2007): *Making Rounds with Oscar: the Extraordinary Gift of an Ordinary Cat.* New York: Hyperion.

Drummond H (1904): *The Lowell Lectures on the Ascent of Man.* Glasgow: Hodder & Stoughton.

Düll T, Düll B (1935): 'Zusammenhange zwischen storungen des erdmagnetismus und haufungen von todesfallen'. *Deutsche Medizinische Wochenschrift*, 61: 95.

Eigen JP (1985): 'Intentionality and insanity: what the eighteenth century juror heard'. *The Anatomy of Madness: Essays in the History of Psychiatry* (volume 2, eds WF Bynum, R Porter, M Shepherd). London: Tavistock. 34–51.

Eisler R (1969): *Man into Wolf: an Anthropological Interpretation of Sadism, Masochism and Lycanthropy.* New York: Green Press.

Esquirol JD (1837/1845): *Mental Maladies: Treatise on Insanity* (translated EK Hunt). Philadelphia: Lea & Blanchard.

Eysenck HJ, Nias DKB (1982): *Astrology: Science or Superstition?* London: Maurice Temple Smith.

Eysenck HJ, Sargent C (1982): *Explaining the Unexplained: Mysteries of the Paranormal.* London: Book Club Associates.

Fairfield L (1954): *Epilepsy.* London: Gerald Duckworth & Co.

Farmer H (1775): *Essay on the Demoniacs of the New Testament.* London: G Robinson.

Farson D, Hall A (1991): *Mysterious Monsters.* London: Bloomsbury.

Financial Times (10/11 July 2010): 'Looney, lunar or simply moonstruck?'

Fitzhugh LC, Hughes LH, Mulvaney DE (1980): *Psychological Reports*, 46: 1261–1262.

Forbes GB, Leno GR (1977): 'Antisocial behavior and lunar activity: a failure to validate the lunacy myth'. *Psychological Reports*, 40: 1309–1310.

Foster RG, Roenneberg T (2008): 'Human responses to the geophysical daily, annual and lunar cycles'. *Current Biology*, 18 (R): 784–794.

Fox HM (1923): 'Lunar periodicity in reproduction'. *Proceedings of the Royal Society of London*, 95: 523–550.

Foucault M (1961) *Madness and Civilization* (translated R Howard).London: Tavistock.

Foucault M (1963/2003) *The Birth of the Clinic: Medical Archaeology* (translated AM Sheridan). London: Routledge.

Freeman H, Stansfield S (eds 2008): *The Impact of the Environment on Psychiatric Disorder*. London: Routledge.

Frey J, Rotton J, Barry T (1979): The effects of the full moon on human behavior: another failure to replicate. *Journal of Psychology*, 103: 159–162.

Friedmann E (1981): Menstrual and lunar cycles. *American Journal of Obstetrics and Gynecology*, 140: 350.

Friedman H, Becker RO (1963): Geomagnetic parameters and psychiatric hospital admissions. *Nature*, 200: 626–628.

Friedman H, Becker RO, Bachman CH (1965): Psychiatric ward behavior and geophysical parameters. *Nature*, 205: 1050–1052.

Friis ML, Lund M (1974): Stress convulsions. *Archives of Neurology*, 31: 155– 59.

Galton F (1879): Generic images. *Proceedings of the Royal Institution*, 9: 9.

Galton F (1879): Psychometric experiments. *Brain*, 2: 149–162.

Garth JM, Lester D (1978): The moon and suicide. *Psychological Reports*, 43: 678.

Garzino SJ (1982): Lunar effects on mental behavior: a defense of the empirical research. *Environment and Behavior*, 14: 395–417.

Geller SH, Shannon HW (1976): The moon, weather and mental hospital contacts: confirmation and explanation of the Transylvania effect. *Journal of Psychiatric Nursing and Mental Health Services*, 14: 13–17.

Gettings F (1990): *The Arkana Dictionary of Astrology*. London: Penguin.

Ghaemi SN (2008): Pluralism in psychiatry: Karl Jaspers on science. *Philosophy, Psychiatry and Psychology*, 14: 57–66.

Gibbs FA, Gibbs EL, Lennox WG (1937): Epilepsy: a paroxysmal cerebral dysrhythmia. *Brain*, 60: 377– 388.

Ghiandoni G, Secli R, Rocchi MBL, Ugolini G (1998): Does lunar position influence the time of delivery? A statistical analysis. *European Journal of Obstetrics and Gynaecology and Reproductive Biology*, 77: 47–50.

Glaser BG, Strauss A (1967): *The Discovery of Grounded Theory*. New York: Aldine de Gruyter.

Goffman E (1961): *Asylums: Essays on the Social Situation of Mental Patients and Other Inmates*. Harmondsworth: Penguin.

Graham TF (1967): *Medieval Minds: Mental Health in the Middle Ages*. London: George Allen & Unwin.

Greenberg G (2010): *Manufacturing Depression: the Secret History of a Modern Disease*. London: Bloomsbury.

Gunn DL, Jenkins PM (1937): Lunar periodicity in *Homo sapiens*. *Nature*, 139: 84.

Guntrip H (1964): *Healing the Sick Mind*. London: George Allen & Unwin.

Guthrie D (1948): *A History of Medicine*. London: Thomas Nelson & Sons.

Hale M (1736): *History of the Pleas of the Crown*. London: E & R Nutt and R Gosling.

Hannam J (2009): *God's Philosophers: How the Medieval World Laid the Foundations of Modern Science*. London: Icon.

Hansen GP (1982): 'Dowsing: a review of experimental research'. *Journal of the Society for Psychical Research*, 51: 343–367.

Harley T (1885): *Moon Lore*. London: Swan Sonnenschein, Le Bas & Lowry.

Hartmann W, Davis D (1975): 'Satellite-sized planetesimals and lunar origin'. *Icarus*, 24 : 504–515.

Haslam J (1809): *Observations on Madness and Melancholy* (2nd edition). London: J Callow.

Healy D (1987): 'Rhythm and blues: neurochemical, neuropharmacological and neuropsychological implications of a hypothesis of a circadian rhythm dysfunction in affective disorders'. *Psychopharmacology*, 93: 271–285.

Healy D (2008): *Mania: a Short History of Bipolar Disorder*. Baltimore: Johns Hopkins University Press.

Hearnshaw LS (1964): *A Short History of British Psychology 1840– 1940*. London: Methuen.

Heider F (1958): *The Psychology of Interpersonal Relations*. New York: John Wiley & Sons.

Henderson DK, Gillespie RD (1950): *Textbook of Psychiatry* (7th edition). London: Oxford University Press.

Hicks-Casey WE, Potter DR (1991): 'Effect of the full moon on developmentally delayed, institutionalized women'. *Perceptual and Motor Skills*, 72: 1375–1380.

Hill D (1981): 'Historical review'. In *Epilepsy and Psychiatry* (ed. EH Reynolds, MR Trimble). Edinburgh: Churchill Livingstone. 1– 11.

Himmelhoch JM (1984): 'Major mood disorders and epileptic changes'. In *Psychiatric Aspects of Epilepsy* (ed. D Blumer). Washington: American Psychiatric Press. 271–291.

Hippocrates (c400BC/1950): *The Medical Works of Hippocrates* (translated J Chadwick, WN Mann). Oxford: Blackwell.

Hodgson GM (2009): 'The great crash of 2008 and the reform of economics'. *Cambridge Journal of Economics*, 33: 1205–1221.

Hoenig J, Lieberman DM (1953): 'The epileptic threshold in schizophrenia'. *Journal of Neurology, Neurosurgery and Psychiatry*, 16: 30–34.

Hone ME (1978): *The Modern Text-Book of Astrology* (revised edition). Romford: LN Fowler.

Hoverson ET (1935): 'The meteorologic factor in mental disease'. *American Journal of Psychiatry*, 92: 131–141.

Hunter R, Macalpine I (1963): *Three Hundred Years of Psychiatry 1535– 1860*. London: Oxford University Press.

Illich I (1976): *Limits to Medicine: Medical Nemesis: The Expropriation of Health*. London: Boyars.

Independent (6 June 2007): 'Police put more officers on beat to tackle "full-moon violence"'.

Iosif A, Ballon B (2005): 'Bad Moon Rising: the persistent belief in lunar connections to madness'. *Canadian Medical Association Journal*, 173: 1498–1500.

James W (1892): 'A plea for psychology as a "natural science"'. *Philosophical Reviews*, 1: 146–153.

Johnson M (2006): The Moon. In *Encyclopedia of Witchcraft: the Western Tradition*. (ed. Golden RM). Santa Barbara, California: ABC-CLIO. 781–783.

Johnstone L (2000): *Users and Abusers of Psychiatry*. London: Routledge.

Jones PK, Jones SL (1977): 'Lunar association with suicide'. *Suicide and Life-Threatening Behavior*, 7: 31– 39.

Jorgenson DO (1981): 'Locus of control and perceived causal influence of the lunar cycle'. *Perceptual and Motor Skills*, 52: 864.

Joshi R, Bharadwaj A, Gallousis S, Matthews R (1998): 'Labor ward workload waxes and wanes with the lunar cycle, myth or reality?' *Primary Care Update for OB/GYNS*, 5: 184.

Jung CG (1911– 1912/1956): 'Symbols of transformation'. In *The Collected Works of CG Jung* (volume 5, translated G Adler, RFC Hull). Princeton: Princeton University Press.

Kahlbaum KL (1863): *Die Gruppirung der psychischen Krankheiten und die Eintheilung der Seelenstoerungen*. Danzig: Kafemann.

Kahlbaum KL (1882): 'Ueber cyklisches Irresein'. *Der Irrenfreund*, 24: 145–157.

Kay RW (1994): 'Geomagnetic storms: association with incidence of depression as measured by hospital admission'. *British Journal of Psychiatry*, 164: 403–409.

Kelly ID, Mazurek K (1983): 'The coherence of claims with scientific theory and "basic limited principles": the case of psychic phenomena'. *Review Journal of Philosophy and Social Sciences*, 8: 82–86.

Kirsch DL (2006): 'Why electromedicine? Harnessing the electrochemical basis of biological processes, electromedicine offers a wide range of applications in the pain area'. *Practical Pain Management*, July/August: 52–54.

Kirsch I (2010): *The Emperor's New Drugs: Exploding the Antidepressant Myth*. Cambridge, Massachusetts: Perseus.

Kitto HDF (1951): *The Greeks*. Harmondsworth: Penguin.

Koestler A (1964): *The Sleepwalkers: A History of Man's Changing Vision of the Universe*. Harmondsworth: Penguin.

Kolbinger HM, Höflich G, Hufnagel A, Müller HJ, Kasper S (1995): 'Transcranial magnetic stimulation (TMS) in the treatment of major depression: a pilot study'. *Human Psychopharmacology: Human and Experimental*, 10: 305–310.

Kolisko L (1936): *The Moon and the Growth of Plants*. Bray-on-Thames: Anthroposophical Agricultural Foundation.

Kollerstrom N, Staudenmaier G (2001): 'Evidence for lunar-sidereal rhythms in crop yield: a review'. *Biological Agriculture and Horticulture*, 19: 247–259.

Koster F (1859): 'Untersuchungen über den Einfluss des Mondes auf das periodische Irresein'. *Allgemeine Zeitschrift für Psychiatrie*, 16: 415–441.

Koster F (1882): *Die Gesetze des periodischen Irreseins und verwandten Nervenstände*. Bonn: Strauss.

Koukopoulus A, Sani G, Koukopoulus AE, Albert MJ, Girardi P, Taterelli R (2006): 'Endogenous and exogenous cyclicity and temperament in bipolar disorder: review, new data and hypotheses'. *Journal of Affective Disorders*, 96: 165–175.

Kraepelin E (1899): *Psychiatrie* (6th edition). Leipzig: Johann Ambrosius Barth.

Kraepelin E (1904): *Psychiatrie* (7th edition). Leipzig: Johann Ambrosius Barth.

Kraepelin E (1913): *Psychiatrie* (8th edition). Leipzig: Johann Ambrosius Barth.

Kuhn TS (1962): *The Structure of Scientific Revolutions*. Chicago: University of Chicago Press.

Kuo J-M, Coakley J, Wood A (2010): 'The lunar moon festival and the dark side of the moon'. *Applied Financial Economics*, 20: 1565–1575.

Langdon-Down M, Brain WR (1929): 'Time of day in relation to convulsions in epilepsy'. *Lancet*, i: 1029-1032.

Laycock T (1843): 'On lunar influence; being a fourth contribution to proleptics'. *Lancet*, ii: 438– 444.

Lee S-H, Kim W, Chung Y-C, Jung K-H, Bahk W-M, Jun T-Y, Kim K-S, George MS, Chae J-H (2005): 'A double blind study showing that two weeks of daily repetitive TMS over the left or right temperoparietal cortex reduces symptoms in patients with schizophrenia who are having treatment-refractory auditory hallucinations'. *Neuroscience Letters*, 376: 177–181.

Leibenluft E (1996): Women with bipolar illness: clinical and research issues. *American Journal of Psychiatry*, 153: 163-173.

Lennox WG (1946): *Science and Seizures: New Light on Epilepsy and Migraine* (2nd edition). New York: Harper & Brothers.

Lester D, Brockopp GW, Priebe K (1969): 'Association between a full moon and completed suicide'. *Psychological Reports*, 25: 598–601.

Leuret F, Mitivié F (1832): *De la Fréquence du Pouls Chez les Aliénes*. Paris: Librairie Médicale de Crochard.

Levy NB (1975): 'On the Journal and the Moon'. *American Journal of Psychiatry*, 132: 85.

Lewin K (1952): *Field Theory in Social Science: Selected Theoretical Papers*. London: Tavistock.

Lewy AJ, Sack RL, Cutler NL, Bauer VK, Hughes RJ (1998): 'Melatonin in circadian phase sleep and mood disorders'. In *Melatonin in Psychiatric and Neoplastic Disorders* (eds M Shafii, SL Shafii). American Psychiatric Press. 81–123.

Liddell DW (1953): 'Observations on epileptic automatisms in a mental hospital population'. *Journal of Mental Science*, 99: 732–748.

Leibenluft E (1996): 'Women with bipolar illness: clinical and research issues'. *American Journal of Psychiatry*, 153: 163–173.

Lennox WG (1946): *Science and Seizures: New Light on Epilepsy and Migraine* (2nd edition). New York: Harper & Brothers.

Lieber AL (1974): 'Comments on "Homicides and the lunar cycle"' (reply). *American Journal of Psychiatry*, 131: 230.

Lieber AL (1978): 'Human aggression and the lunar synodic cycle'. *Journal of Clinical Psychiatry*, 39: 385–393.

Lieber AL (1978): *The Lunar Effect: Biological Tides and Human Emotions*. Garden City, New York: Doubleday.

Lieber A (1996*): How the Moon Affects You*. Mamaroneck, New York: Hastings House.

Lieber AL, Sherin CR (1972): 'Homicides and the lunar cycle: toward a theory of lunar influence on human emotional disturbance'. *American Journal of Psychiatry*, 129: 69–74.

Lilienfeld DM (1969): 'Lunar effect on mental illness'. *American Journal of Psychiatry*, 129: 101–106.

Luce GG (ed, 1970): *Biological Rhythms in Psychiatry and Medicine*. Washington DC: United States Government Printing Office.

Mädler JH (1837): 'Über den Einfluss des Mondes auf die Witterung'. In *Der Mond nach seinen kosmischen und individuellen Verhältnissen, oder Allgemeine vergleichende Selenographie* (eds W Beer, JH Mädler). Berlin. 154–168.

Marcuse FL (1959): *Hypnosis: Fact and Fiction*. Harmondsworth: Penguin.

Matthew, 17:15. *Holy Bible – King James' Version* (1611/2008). London: Collins.

Maudsley H (1873) *Body and Mind*. London: Macmillan.

Mayer-Gross W, Slater E, Roth M (1955): *Clinical Psychiatry*. London: Cassell & Company.

McCrae N (2009): 'Non-electrical shock therapies'. In *Electroconvulsive and Neuromodulation Therapies* (ed. C Swartz). Cambridge University Press. 17–43.

Mead R (1746): 'Treatise concerning the influence of the Sun and Moon upon human bodies, and the diseases thereby produced'. In *The Medical Works of Richard Mead*. Dublin: Thomas Ewing.

Menaker W, Menaker A (1959): 'Lunar periodicity in human reproduction: a likely unit of biological time'. *American Journal of Obstetrics and Gynecology*, 77: 905–914.

Menzies IEP (1960): 'The functioning of social systems as a defence against anxiety: a report on a study of the nursing service of a general hospital'. *Human Relations*, 13: 95–121.

Merleau-Ponty M (1945/1962): *Phenomenology of Perception* (translated C Smith). London: Routledge.

Merritt HH, Putman TJ (1938): 'A new series of anticonvulsant drugs tested by experiments on animals'. *Archives of Neurology and Psychiatry*, 39: 1003–1015.

Michelson L, Wilson J, Michelson J (1979): 'Investigation of periodicity in crisis intervention calls over an eight year span'. *Psychological Reports*, 45:420–422.

Mills CA (1934): 'Suicides and homicides in their relation to weather changes'. *American Journal of Psychiatry*, 91: 669–677.

Molland AG (1968): 'The geometrical background to the Merton School'. *British Journal for the History of Science*, 4: 108–125.

Moncrieff J(2001): 'Are antidepressants overrated? A review of methodological problems in antidepressant trials'. *Journal of Nervous and Mental Disease*, 189: 288–295.

Moore P (1992): *Fireside Astronomy*. Chichester: John Wiley & Sons.

Myers DE (1995): 'Gravitational effects of the period of high tides and the new moon on lunacy'. *Journal of Emergency Medicine*, 13: 529–532.

Neal RD, Colledge M (2000): 'The effect of the full moon on general practice consultation rates'. *Family Practice*, 17: 472–474.

Nishumara T, Fakushima M (2009): 'Why animals respond to the full moon: magnetic hypothesis'. *Bioscience Hypotheses*, 2: 399–401.

Nunez S, Perez Mundez L, Aguirre-Jaime A (2002): 'Moon cycles and violent behaviours: myth or fact?' *European Journal of Emergency Medicine*, 9: 127–130.

O'Donahue WT, Lilienfeld SO, Fowler KA (2007): 'Science is an essential safeguard against human error'. In *The Great Ideas of Clinical Science: 17 Principles that every Mental Health Professional should Understand* (eds SO Lilenfeld, WT O'Donahue). New York: Routledge. 1–27.

Oliven JF (1943): 'Moonlight and nervous disorders: a historical study'. *American Journal of Psychiatry*, 99: 579–584.

Osborn RD (1968): 'The moon and mental hospital: an investigation of one area of folklore'. *Journal of Psychiatric Nursing and Mental Health Services*, 6: 88–93.

Ossenkopp K-P, Ossenkopp MD (1973): 'Self-inflicted injuries and the lunar cycle: a preliminary report'. *Journal of Interdisciplinary Cycle Research*, 4: 337–348.

Otis LP, Kuo ECY (1984): 'Extraordinary beliefs among students in Singapore andCanada'. *Journal of Psychology*, 116: 215–226.

Owen C, Tarantello C, Jones M, Tennant C (1998): 'Lunar cycles and violent behaviour'. *Australian and New Zealand Journal of Psychiatry*, 32: 496–499.

Panda S, Hogenesch JB, Kay SA (2002): 'Circadian rhythms from flies to human'. *Nature*, 417: 329–335.

Park K (2009): 'Myth 5: That the medieval church prohibited human dissection'. In *Galileo goes to Jail and Other Myths about Science and Religion* (ed. RL Numbers). New York: Harvard University Press.

Partonen T, Haukka J, Viilo K, Hakko H, Pirkola S, Isometsä J, Särkioja T, Väisänen E, Räsänen P (2004): 'Cyclic time patterns of death from suicide in northern Finland'. *Journal of Affective Disorders*, 78: 11–19.

Patch CJL (1934): *A Manual of Mental Diseases: a Textbook for Students and Practitioners in India*. London: Baillière Tindall & Cox.

Patey EH (1978): *All in Good Faith*. Oxford: Mowbrays.

Pearson K (1911) *The Grammar of Science* (3rd edition). London: A & C Black.

Perper JA, Cina SJ (2010): *When Doctors Kill: Who, Why and How*. New York: Springer.

Persinger MSA, Psych C (1995): 'Sudden unexpected death in epileptics following sudden, intense increases in geomagnetic activity: prevalence of effect and potential mechanisms'. *International Journal of Biometeorology* 38: 180–187.

Peterson WF (1947): *Man, Weather, Sun*. Springfield, Illinois. Charles C Thomas.

Pinel P (1806/1962): *Treatise on Insanity* (2nd edition, translated DD Davies). New York: Hafner.

Plato (c380BC/1955): *The Republic* (translated D Lee). Harmondsworth: Penguin.

Pochobradsky J (1974): 'Independence of human menstruation on lunar phases and days of the week'. *American Journal of Obstetrics & Gynecology*, 118: 1136–1138.

Pokorny AD (1964): 'Moon phase, suicide and homicide'. *American Journal of Psychiatry*, 121: 66–67.

Pokorny AD, David F, Harberson W (1964): 'Suicide, suicide attempts, and weather'. *American Journal of Psychiatry*, 120: 377–381.

Pokorny AD, Jachimczyk J (1974): 'The questionable relationship between homicides and the lunar cycle'. *American Journal of Psychiatry*, 131: 827–829.

Polychronopoulus P, Argyriou AA, Sirrou V, Huliara V, Aplada M, Gouzis P, Economou A, Terzis E, Chroni E (2006): 'Lunar phases and seizure occurrence: just an ancient legend?' *Neurology*, 66: 1442–1443.

Popper KR (1959): The *Logic of Scientific Discovery*. London: Hutchinson & Co.

Raison CL, Klein HM, Steckler M (1999): 'The moon and madness reconsidered'. *Journal of Affective Disorders*, 53: 99–106.

Rajna P, Veres J (1993): 'Correlations between night sleep duration and seizure frequency in temporal lobe epilepsy'. *Epilepsia*, 34: 574–579.

Raps A , Soupel E, Shimshoni M (1991):' Solar activity and admissions of psychiatric inpatients, relations and possible implications on seasonality'. *Israeli Journal of Psychiatry and Related Sciences*, 28: 72–80.

Ravitz LJ (1962): 'History, measurement, and applicability of periodic changes in the electromagnetic field in health and disease'. *Annals of the New York Academy of Science*, 98: 1144–1201.

Reppert SM, Gegear RJ, Merlin C (2010): 'Navigational mechanisms of migrating monarch butterflies'. *Trends in Neurosciences*, 9: 399–406.

Rodger H (1809): *A Small Treatise of Astronomy*. Kilmarnock: H & S Crawford.

Rogers ME (1970): *An Introduction to the Theoretical Basis of Nursing*. Philadelphia: FA Davis.

Rogers TD, Masterton G, McGuire R (1991): 'Parasuicide and the lunar cycle'. *Psychological Medicine*, 21: 393–397.

Röösli M, Jüni P, Braun-Fahrländer C, Brinkhof MWG, Low N, Egger M (2006): Sleepless night, the moon is bright: longitudinal study of lunar phase and sleep. *Journal of Sleep Research*, 15: 149-153.

Rorsch PJ (2009): 'Bioelectromagnetic and subtle energy medicine: the interface between mind and matter'. *Annals of the New York Academy of Science*, 1172: 297–311.

Rosenhan DL (1982) 'On being sane in insane places'. In *Social Research Ethics* (ed. M Bulmer). New York: Holmes & Meier. 15-37.

Rotter JB (1966): 'Generalised expectancies for internal versus external control of reinforcement'. *Psychological Monographs*, 80: 169–214.

Rotton J, Kelly IW (1985a): 'Much ado about the full moon: a meta-analysis of lunar-lunacy research'. *Psychological Bulletin*, 97: 286–306.

Rotton J, Kelly IW (1985b) 'A scale for assessing belief in lunar effects: reliability and concurrent validity'. *Psychological Reports*, 57: 239–245.

Rotton J, Kelly IW, Elortegui P (1986): 'Assessing belief in lunar effects: known-groups validation'. *Psychological Reports*, 59: 171–174.

Rovang D (2006): 'When reason reigns: madness, passions and sovereignty in late 18th-century England'. *History of Psychiatry*, 17: 23–44.

Rüegg S, Hunziker P, Marsch S, Schindler C (2008): 'Association of environmental factors with the onset of status epilepticus'. *Epilepsy and Behavior*, 12: 66–73.

Russell B (1952/1994): *The Impact of Science on Society*. London: Routledge.

Russell GW, Dua M (1983): 'Lunar influences on human aggression'. *Social Behavior and Personality*, 11: 41–44.

Ryan J, Thomas F (1980): *The Politics of Mental Handicap*. Harmondsworth: Penguin.

Sábato MAL, de Melo LFB, Magni EMV, Young RJ, Coelho CM (2006): 'A note on the effect of the full moon on the activity of wild maned wolves, *Chysocyon brachyurus*'. *Behavioural Processes*, 73: 228–230.

Sarton G (1939): 'Lunar influences on living things'. *Isis*, 30: 495–507.

Savage GH, Goodall E (1907): *Insanity and Allied Neuroses: A Practical and Clinical Manual*. London: Cassell.

Schultz PH, Hermalyn B, Colaprete A, Ennico K, Shirley M, Marshall WS (2010): 'The LCROSS Cratering Experiment'. *Science*, 330: 468–472.

Schumacher EF (1977): *A Guide for the Perplexed*. London: Abacus.

Scott D (1969): *About Epilepsy*. London: Duckworth.

Scull AT (1979): *Museums of Madness: the Social Organization of Insanity in 19th Century England*. London: Allen Lane.

Sendak M (1963): *Where the Wild Things Are*. New York: Harper.

Senge P (1990): *The Fifth Discipline*. New York: Doubleday.

Shakespeare W (1604/1996). *Othello*. Act V, scene II. *Complete Works of William Shakespeare*. Wordsworth.

Shankar D, Unnikrishnan PM (ed. 2004): *Challenging the Indian Medical Heritage*. New Delhi: Foundation Books.

Shapiro JL, Streiner DL, Gray AL, Williams NL, Soble C (1970): 'The moon and mental illness: a failure to confirm the Transylvania effect'. *Perceptual and Motor Skills*, 30: 827–830.

Shepherd JP (1990): 'Violent crime in Bristol: an A & E perspective'. *British Journal of Criminology*, 30: 289–305.

Skultans V (1979): *English Madness: Ideas on Insanity 1580–1890*. London: Routledge & Kegan Paul.

Solomon RC (1993): *The Passions: Emotions and the Meaning of Life*. Indianapolis: Hackett.

Stanton AH, Schwartz MS (1954): *The Mental Hospital: a Study of Institutional Participation in Psychiatric Illness and Treatment*. New York: Basic Books.

Stevens JR (1998): 'Seizure or psychosis: alternative brain responses to the physiological events of puberty, the reproductive period, brain injury or malformation'. In *Forced Normalization and Alternative Psychoses of Epilepsy* (eds MR Trimble, B Schmitz). Petersfield: Wrightson Biomedical. 121–141.

Stolov HL, Cameron AGW (1964): Variations of geomagnetic activity with lunar phase. *Journal of Geophysical Research*, 69: 4975-4982.

Sunday Times (2 January 2011): 'Atheists: a dying breed as nature favours faithful'.

Swinscow D (1951): 'Some suicide statistics'. *British Medical Journal*, i: 1417–1423.

Symonds RL, Williams P (1976): 'Seasonal variations in the incidence of mania'. *British Journal of Psychiatry*, 129: 45–48.

Szasz T (2007): *Coercion as Cure: a Critical History of Psychiatry*. Piscataway, New Jersey: Transaction.

Takezaki H, Hanaoka M (1971): 'The use of carbamaepine (Tegretol) in the control of manic-depressive psychosis and other manic-depressive states'. *Clinical Psychiatry*, 13: 173–183.

Tasso J, Miller E (1976): 'The effects of the full moon on human behavior'. *Journal of Psychology*, 93: 81–83.

Taylor LJ, Diespecker DD (1972): 'Moon phases and suicide attempts in Australia'. *Psychological Reports*, 31: 110.

Temkin O (1971): *The Falling Sickness* (2nd edition). Baltimore: John Hopkins Press.

Templer DI, Veleber DM (1980): 'The moon and madness: a comprehensive perspective'. *Journal of Clinical Psychology*, 36: 865–868.

Terra-Bustamante VC, Scorza CA, de Albuquerque M, Sakamoto AC, Machado HR, Arida RM, Cavalheiro EA, Scorza FA (2009): 'Does the lunar phase have an effect on sudden unexpected death in epilepsy?' *Epilepsy and Behavior*, 14: 404–406.

Thiel R (1958):*And There Was Light: The Discovery of the Universe* (translated R Winston, C Winston). André Deutsch.

Toofani H, Musavi SA (2001): 'Lunar phases and overdose attempted suicide'. *Iranian Journal of Psychiatry and Clinical Psychology*, 6.

Trapp CE (1937): 'Lunacy and the moon'. *American Journal of Psychiatry*, 94: 339–342.

Treasure G (1985): *The Making of Modern Europe 1648–1780*. London: Methuen.

Turner EH, Matthews AM, Linardatos E, Tell RA, Rosenthal R (2008): 'Selective publication of antidepressant trials and its influence on apparent efficacy'. *New England Journal of Medicine*, 358: 252–260.

Tylor EB (1873): *Primitive Culture*. London: Watts.

Vance DE (1995): 'Belief in lunar effects on human behavior'. *Psychological Reports*, 76: 32–34.

Veyne P (1988): *Did the Greeks Believe in their Myths? An Essay on the Constitutive Imagination* (translated P Wissing). Chicago: University of Chicago Press.

Völgyesi F (1935): *A Message to the Neurotic World* (translated B Balogh). London: Hutchinson & Co.

von Bertalanffy, L (1950): 'An outline of general system theory'. *British Journal for the Philosophy of Science*, 1: 134–165.

Voracek M, Loibl LM, Kapusta ND, Niederkrotenhaler T, Dervic K, Sonneck G (2008): 'Not carried away by the moonlight shadow: no evidence for associations between suicide occurrence and lunar phase among more than 65000 suicide cases in Austria, 1970–2006'. *Wiener Klinische Wochenschrift*, 120: 343–349.

Walters E, Markley RP, Tiffany DW (1975): 'Lunacy: a type I error?' *Journal of Abnormal Psychology*, 84: 715–717.

Webster C (1979): 'Alchemical and Paracelsian medicine'. In *Health, Medicine and Mortality in the Sixteenth Century* (ed. C Webster). 301–334.

Wehr TA (1989): 'Seasonal affective disorder: a historical overview'. In *Seasonal Affective Disorders and Phototherapy* (eds NE Rosenthal, MC Blehar). New York: Guilford Press. 11–32.

Wehr TA (1992): 'Improvement of depression and triggering of mania by sleep deprivation'. *Journal of the American Medical Association*, 267: 548–551.

Weiskott GN, Tipton GB (1975): 'Moon phases and state hospital admissions'. *Psychological Reports*, 37: 486–490.

Wetterburg L (1998): 'Melatonin in adult depression'. In *Melatonin in Psychiatric and Neoplastic Disorders* (eds M Shafii, SL Shafii). American Psychiatric Press. 43–79.

White EW (1900): 'Epilepsy associated with insanity'. *Journal of Mental Science*, 46: 73–79.

White WA (1914): 'Moon myth in medicine'. *Psychoanalytic Review*, 1: 241–256.

Whitehouse D (2003): *The Moon: A Biography*. London: Headline.

Wilkinson G, Piccinelli M, Roberts S, Micciolo R, Fry J (1997): 'Lunar cycle and consultations for anxiety and depression in general practice'. *International Journal of Social Psychiatry*, 43: 29–34.

Wilson JE, Tobacyk JJ (1989): 'Lunar phases and crisis center telephone calls'. *Journal of Social Psychology*, 130: 47–51.

Wiltschko R, Wiltschko W (2006): 'Magnetoreception'. *Bioessays*, 28: 157–168.

Winslow F (1867) *Light: its Influence on Life and Health*. London: Longmans & Co.

Winstead DK, Schwartz BD, Bertrand WE (1981): 'Biorhythms: fact or superstition?' *American Journal of Psychiatry*, 138: 1188–1192.

Wolf P, Trimble MR (1985): 'Biological antagonism and epileptic psychosis'. *British Journal of Psychiatry*, 146: 272–276.

World Health Organization (2002): *The World Health Report 2002: Reducing Risks, Promoting Healthy Life*. Geneva: World Health Organization.

Yin RK (1994): *Case Study Research: Design and Methods* (2nd edition). Thousand Oaks, California: Sage.

Zeitzer JN, Dijk D-J, Kronauer RE, Brown EN, Czeisler CA (2000): 'Sensitivity of the human circadian pacemaker to nocturnal light: melatonin, phase-resetting and suppression'. *Journal of Physiology*, 526: 695-702.

Zilboorg G (1941): *A History of Medical Psychology*. New York: WW Norton.

Index